This is a comprehensive overview of hypertension incorporates conventional medical wisdom as well up-to-date thinking regarding the important role of stress. Readers will find clear explanations of hypertension: its causes, deleterious effects on the body, and an explanation of the types of drugs used to treat it. But they will also learn about our growing understanding of the important contribution of stress hormones and will learn some simple techniques to engage their hearts and brains to restore inner equilibrium and calmness. This will be useful for anyone who wants to understand hypertension and the range of options available to address it.

—Kenneth M. Riff, MD, executive director of the Hawaii
Heart Brain Center at North Hawaii Community Hospital

As this concise but meaty book emphasizes, hypertension is a major cause of death and disability. It is aptly called "the silent killer" because patients may have no symptoms until it produces significant damage. Although there are numerous antihypertensive drugs, there is no algorithm that guarantees which will work best in any given patient and many have serious side effects. In contrast, the HeartMath® approach is completely safe and its efficacy has been demonstrated in years of cutting-edge research on heart rate variability feedback.

—Paul Rosch, MD, president of the American Institute
of Stress

D0250247

Connecting the mind, body, and emotions, Heartmath offers a quickly learned, scientifically validated approach to decreasing stress and impacting cardiac risk factors such as high blood pressure, diabetes, arrhythmia, and chest pain. Everyone needs to learn these techniques.

—Mimi Guarneri, MD, FACC, medical director of the Scripps
Center for Integrative Medicine

The holistic approach to hypertension described in this book is user-friendly for patients of different ages. It addresses the essential bio-behavioral nature of the problem directly, with ideas to heal and balance body and mind.

—Timothy P. Culbert, MD, medical director, integrative medicine and cultural care, at Children's Hospitals and Clinics of Minnesota

Wilson and Childre present an up-to-date, highly readable, and comprehensive approach to managing high blood pressure. Using a combination of evidence-based clinical recommendations (medications, exercise, and diet) together with scientifically validated HeartMath® tools, the authors clearly and concisely explain the key role of the heart-brain connection ("heart intelligence") in the management of hypertension. If you have hypertension, this book is a must read. If your blood pressure is normal but your life is stressful (let's be honest — whose life is not?), I am convinced that combining HeartMath® tools with a good diet and adequate exercise can help you achieve emotional balance and optimal health.

—Alan P. Feren, MD, president of Feren Healthcare Insights, LLC, and former chief medical officer of Sutter Health Partners

One third of Americans have high blood pressure. It is therefore likely that you or someone you love has this health problem (and may not even know it). Do you know how high blood pressure happens? Wilson and Childre teach us not only the causes of high blood pressure but how to take care of it, with reduced medication or no medication at all. All Americans should read this book.

—Lee Lipsenthal, MD, ABHM, heart disease researcher and president of the American Board of Holistic Medicine

The increasingly complex and ambiguous business world we now live in, and the speed at which this world can change, can result in maladaptive physiological responses in people. This often leads to a stress response mechanism which can result in sustained hypertension, which in its initial stages produces no symptoms. If sustained too long, it can result in profound and serious future health effects. Whilst medication, with all its potential side effects, has been the mainstay of treatment for several years, HeartMath's research has been instrumental in demonstrating the role of certain emotional states in our stress response mechanisms. HeartMath® philosophy and tools have shown that by influencing these emotional states and their associated physiological mechanisms often responsible for hypertension, patients can take control and positively improve their physiology. This can result in preventing hypertension at an early stage, avoiding or delaying medication, or significantly reducing the quantity and dose of already prescribed antihypertensive medication.

—Tony Yardley-Jones, MD, Ph.D., specialist in occupational medicine at Chelsea & Westminster, London, UK, and director of occupational health at the Royal Berkshire Hospital, Reading, UK

Stress and its consequences remain major hurdles as people search for ways to improve quality of life and reduce susceptibility to illness. Wilson and Childre have put together a well-referenced, scientifically supported, novel approach to the management of one of our nation's biggest killers — hypertension. Knowing how vulnerable we are to developing high blood pressure is what makes the HeartMath® approach so interesting and helpful. Having tools that can positively influence our responses to the stresses of daily life is critical in the battle against heart disease and stroke. Taking charge of our life stressors has great potential to decrease not only our blood pressure but reduce our susceptibility to other stress-related health problems. Enjoy the book and take the message 'to heart.'

—Kathy Berra, MSN, ANP, FAAN, past president of the American Association of Cardiovascular and Pulmonary Rehabilitation Cardiovascular Medicine and Coronary Interventions, Redwood City, CA

While there are hundreds of books on controlling high blood pressure, The HeartMath® Approach to Managing Hypertension *clearly stands out as breakthrough work. Unlike any authors before them, Wilson and Childre have clearly recognized the role stress plays in elevating blood pressure and have developed scientifically-proven techniques for reducing stress and, thus, lowering blood pressure. This comprehensive book explains the causes of hypertension, the pros and cons of medications used to treat the condition, and looks at both conventional and alternative treatments. But most importantly, what you learn in* The HeartMath® Approach to Managing Hypertension *works! And that is a major step forward.*

—Charles B. Inlander, president of People's Medical Society

This book not only discusses the link between stress and high blood pressure, but also serves as a great resource for how to break stress and its toxic effects in all people — not just those with hypertension. As the CEO of a large hospital, I am wholly supportive of the HeartMath® methodology to reduce stress in the workplace and in our daily lives. I have seen it work in my organization. The pace of our culture has increased dramatically over the past few decades, and if we do not take control of the issues that cause stress in our lives, we will not be able to perform the important services expected of us in the health care industry.

—Mary M. White, chief executive officer of the Swedish Medical Center, Denver, CO

This is a work that is informative and highly readable. It addresses a significant public health problem in a straightforward and practical way. You can feel the passion and caring put forth by these dedicated professionals. I can highly recommend it to anyone in the health care field as well as individuals afflicted by this chronic illness.

—Nick Hilger, senior vice president of strategic development for United Healthcare

HeartMath®

Approach to Managing

Hypertension

The Proven, Natural Way to Lower Your Blood Pressure

Bruce C. Wilson, MD • Doc Childre

New Harbinger Publications, Inc.

Publisher's Note

This publication is designed to provide accurate and authoritative information in regard to the subject matter covered. It is sold with the understanding that the publisher is not engaged in rendering psychological, financial, legal, or other professional services. If expert assistance or counseling is needed, the services of a competent professional should be sought.

Care has been taken to confirm the accuracy of the information presented and to describe generally accepted practices. However, the authors, editors, and publisher are not responsible for errors or omissions or for any consequences from application of the information in this book and make no warranty, express or implied, with respect to the contents of the publication.

Some drugs and medical devices presented in this publication may have Food and Drug Administration (FDA) clearance for limited use in restricted research settings. It is the responsibility of the health care provider to ascertain the FDA status of each drug or device planned for use in their clinical practice.

HeartMath, Heart Lock-In, and Inner Quality Management are registered trademarks of the Institute of HeartMath. Quick Coherence and Freeze-Framer are registered trademarks of Quantum Intech, Inc.

Distributed in Canada by Raincoast Books

Copyright © 2006 by Doc Childre and Bruce C. Wilson, MD
New Harbinger Publications, Inc.
5674 Shattuck Avenue
Oakland, CA 94609
www.newharbinger.com

Cover design by Amy Shoup; Text design by Tracy Carlson;
Acquired by Jess O'Brien; Edited by Amy Scott

Library of Congress Cataloging-in-Publication Data

Wilson, Bruce C.
  The Heartmath approach to managing hypertension : the proven, natural way to lower your blood pressure / Bruce C. Wilson and Doc Childre.
       p. cm.
  ISBN-13: 978-1-57224-471-9
  ISBN-10: 1-57224-471-2
  1. Hypertension—Alternative treatment. 2. Hypertension—Psychosomatic aspects. I. Childre, Doc Lew, 1945- II. Title.
RC685.H8W527 2006
616.1'3206—dc22

                                    2006031464

All Rights Reserved
Printed in the United States of America

09 08 07

10 9 8 7 6 5 4 3 2

Dedication

This book is dedicated to all people who want to take more personal responsibility for their own health, learn about exciting research that links stress and emotions to disease (high blood pressure in particular), and use simple proven tools to help lower blood pressure.

Using HeartMath tools has the capacity to change your life in many ways. It has been the goal of the entire Heart-Math team, since 1990, to understand how physical responses to multiple stress-producing events in a complex world impact health and how people might change those responses to achieve better health and well-being—and eventually, a better planet.

Contents

Foreword

Cardiovascular disease is the leading cause of morbidity and mortality in the United States today. Although men with heart trouble have attracted attention for years, cardiovascular disease also claims 500,000 women's lives per year, more than all cancers combined. Yet despite these staggering statistics, cardiovascular disease is totally preventable.

Western society suffers from what can best be described as diseases of excess. These include diabetes, hypertension, gout, and hyperlipidemia, all of which are major risk factors for heart disease and stroke. Unfortunately, we live in a society that has many addictions, including food, tobacco, alcohol, and even stress. These addictions are frequently the underlying cause for many of these medical problems.

To heal the heart and prevent cardiovascular disease, a mind, body, and spirit approach is truly needed. Our physical bodies are greatly affected by the food we eat, the amount that we exercise, and the length of time that we sleep. We must also recognize that the human heart is deeply affected by emotions such as anger and hostility. The way we live our lives and who we share our lives with can have profound consequences on our emotional and physical health.

Hypertension is one of the leading causes of heart attack and stroke. It is appropriately referred to as "the silent killer," since many people have hypertension and don't know it. Treating hypertension, like treating all of the other risk factors for cardiovascular disease, requires a multidisciplinary approach. This means getting to the underlying cause of the problem and making the necessary changes to reset the body toward health, which comes from the Greek word for "wholeness."

Hippocrates said, "let food be your medicine," and no truer words have been spoken for the prevention of cardiovascular disease. Each year, 300,000 Americans die from a combination of poor diet and inactivity. We now know that 30 to 50 percent of individuals with hypertension will be "salt sensitive." This means that the simple restriction of salt in the diet, to as low as 1,500 milligrams per day, can have a profound effect on blood pressure. Many people are shocked to learn of the amount of sodium in common food items such as cheese, pickles, and soup and items high in saturated fat such as bacon and ham. I teach my patients to shop around the periphery of the supermarket and focus on fresh fruits and vegetables, avoiding canned items whenever possible.

Any nutrition program must be accompanied by proper exercise. The benefits of exercise are enormous, and include a decrease in body weight, blood sugar, and triglyceride levels. Exercise will also lower blood pressure and decrease the level of stress hormones such as adrenaline and cortisol. In addition, exercise helps us to sleep better at night and should be the first treatment for insomnia. The combination of diet and exercise can have profound effects on the body. We know from the Lyon Heart Study that cardiovascular event rates were decreased by 70 percent in individuals taught to eat more fruit, beans, vegetables, and fish. We also know that men and women who exercise modestly, such as walking 1.5 miles per day, can decrease their risk of cardiovascular death by 50 percent. There is no known medication that can achieve these results, and this is why all of my patients at the Scripps Center for Integrative Medicine receive a prescription for diet and exercise.

Although diet and exercise are important first steps in improving blood pressure as well as decreasing blood sugar, weight, and cholesterol, they are just a piece of the puzzle. We know from the American Institute of Stress that 75 to 90 percent of all visits to health care providers result from stress-related disorders. As a cardiologist, when I first heard this statistic I thought it must be too high. However, after carefully assessing the reasons why people come to see me in my practice, I quickly realized that this number was right on. Stress leads to the release of hormones originally evolved to assist us in an emergency situation. For example, if you have an auto accident and are bleeding, your body produces adrenaline to keep the blood pressure up, increase the heart rate to pump more blood to your vital organs, and constrict the blood vessels to minimize blood loss. The stress hormones should absolutely be released in a state of true emergency such as this, because they can be lifesaving.

The problem is that we have evolved to a point in our culture where we are producing these stress hormones on a daily basis, and in response to events that don't even come close to being life threatening. Meeting deadlines, rushing through traffic, and answering cell phones, e-mails, and faxes is just a short list of how our society is accelerating. The end result is that our body senses a threat much in the same way as if we were bleeding or being chased by a tiger. Stress hormones pour into our systems, the end result being an increase in heart rate and occasionally disturbances in heart rhythm, as well as an increase in blood pressure, blood sugar, and even cholesterol levels.

Many of the cardiac medications given on a daily basis are designed to block stress hormones. Adrenaline, for example, which increases heart rate, constricts blood vessels, and raises blood pressure, is blocked by beta-blocker drugs. This class of medication is given to lower heart rate and blood pressure, and prevent heart attack. It is no surprise that these medications also reduce the negative effect of adrenaline on the heart. Aldosterone, like adrenaline, is a stress hormone that raises blood pressure by causing salt and water retention. Inhibition of aldosterone is one of the targets achieved by initiating diuretic therapy (water pills) in individuals with known hypertension or congestive heart failure.

The intriguing question is this: How can we change our responses to stress and still maintain a system that will protect us in life-threatening situations? Many lifestyle-change programs are successful at helping individuals to master the stress response; yoga, meditation, tai chi, and progressive muscle relaxation are just a few of the techniques that can be beneficial in this area. The HeartMath program described in this book by Dr. Wilson and Doc Childre offers a unique opportunity in the arena of stress management because these techniques can be learned quickly and applied immediately. Being able to recognize a stressful situation and taking a quick time-out to begin a simple breathing technique while shifting your emotional attitude has a profound effect on the nervous system. It changes your physiology from a "fight-or-flight" stimulated state to one of calm and clarity. The simple end result is a decrease in stress hormone production with a resultant decrease in blood pressure and heart rate.

As you practice the HeartMath techniques found in this book, you will learn how to quickly move from a hyper-agitated state to one of wider perspective and positive attitude. You will improve not only your physiology but your cognitive brain function as well. HeartMath is powerful medicine.

—Mimi Guarneri, MD, FACC
  Medical Director
  Scripps Center for Integrative Medicine
  La Jolla, California

Acknowledgments

Stress as a cause or a contributor to physical ailments is not a new concept. Long before the science of medicine was developed, it was understood that emotions and outside pressures could have significant health consequences. In the 1930s Professor Hans Selye at the University of Montreal began to scientifically study stress. His work opened many doors. Beatrice and John Lacey made great advances in the 1970s when they observed a link between the heartbeat and brain function.

As we enter the twenty-first century, new fields of scientific exploration have emerged. Psychoneuroimmunology studies the connection between emotions, the nervous system, and the immune system. Neurocardiology examines the electrical, chemical, and electromagnetic communication between the heart, the brain, and the rest of the nervous system.

We are greatly indebted to all those who have pushed and pulled, stayed up late at night and scribbled on napkins, asking questions and searching for answers to how the human system works and how health and well-being can be improved. Our immense gratitude goes to our own research team, headed by Dr. Rollin McCraty, which includes Mike

Atkinson, Dana Tomasino, Jackie Waterman, and Ray Bradley. Guidance and query from the Scientific Advisory Board at the Institute of HeartMath is also greatly appreciated.

Special thanks goes to Dr. Mimi Guarneri, author of *The Heart Speaks*, cardiologist, and medical director of the Scripps Center for Integrative Medicine in La Jolla, California, for her enthusiastic support of HeartMath and willingness to write the foreword to this book.

Finally, we are grateful to Dr. Deborah Rozman for her boundless commitment, energy, and oversight in getting this book completed; Amy Scott, who also gave us wonderful editorial assistance; and Regina Valuch, medical librarian at Columbia Hospital in Milwaukee, Wisconsin, who deserves special commendation for her skill and speed in producing reference material.

Introduction

Bruce C. Wilson, MD, FACC

According to the National Institutes of Health, the number of adults with high blood pressure has risen dramatically over the last ten years. In 1990, approximately one in four adults in the United States had hypertension. In 2000, it was about one in three Americans, or sixty-five million people over the age of eighteen, with elevated blood pressure. This represents a 30 percent jump—a very worrisome trend, to be sure.

This is a big issue. High blood pressure is a major risk factor for the development of heart disease, including coronary artery disease (the number-one killer of Americans) and congestive heart failure (the number-one cause for hospital admission in people over the age of sixty-five). It is also a major risk factor for stroke and kidney damage.

By now, most people know that the population is not only growing older, but growing fatter as well. Obesity is an epidemic in the United States and other countries, and efforts are underway to reevaluate patterns of eating and exercise. Being overweight is a very strong predictor of the development of high blood pressure, in addition to many other diseases, so it must be attacked on this front as well. It is said that if your belly is the first thing to pass through the door as you enter a room, you're in trouble.

As a society, we must face the music and stop this rapid increase in the number of people who have hypertension by preventing it, not just treating it. And it is preventable in many cases.

Prevention and Control

As far as your number of birthdays goes, doctors know that if you are fifty-five and you do not have hypertension, there's still a 90 percent chance you will develop it sometime in your life if you don't do something to prevent it. When you are young, fifty-five sounds ancient. But when you get to fifty-five, most feel they have many more years to go. People are living much longer these days. The average life span now is in the upper seventies and many live far longer. If the vast majority of people over fifty-five will develop high blood pressure at some time, they must start early if they are to prevent high blood pressure and all of its health-deteriorating consequences.

Take obesity, for example. Because being overweight is such a strong predictor for the development of hypertension, and because it has become so common in young people, guidelines have been published by the National Heart, Lung, and Blood Institute for physicians to help children and adolescents as well as adults adopt heart-healthy eating habits, lessen their intake of salt, and exercise more.

If you can't prevent high blood pressure and have to treat it instead, then it's better to do so without unwanted side effects. Over the years, great progress has been made in the treatment of hypertension. Today's culture seems to want to take a pill and make everything right. However, many of the medications now used to treat high blood pressure, while effective, cause other health problems in a number of people taking them. Many people need to be concerned about possible side effects, especially when multiple medications are necessary.

Natural Help

There has been a major shift over the years to try to use more "natural" therapies. Indeed, the understanding that the human body has a great capacity to heal itself has been the subject of many areas of research.

In this book we will first examine the current understanding of high blood pressure, its causes, and the problems it can create. Then we'll discuss the pharmacologic treatments of hypertension. We will see how various classes of medications work, as well as review some of the side effects that can be experienced by people taking them. The middle section of the book will explore the biology of stress and the many ways it can harm you, even though your body's response to stress (physical threats) was originally designed to help you. Finally, the chapters toward the end will be your education in the HeartMath approach to lowering blood pressure by interfering with this built-in stress response. Lowering your blood pressure while reducing the stress in your life sounds like a real bargain, doesn't it?

The HeartMath Approach

We will open the door to a recent and very exciting area of research—one which examines how the heart communicates with the brain as well as the rest of the body—and how this has resulted in an effective and proven natural treatment that has lowered blood pressure for many.

Findings at the Institute of HeartMath in California have allowed us to probe deeply into this area, which is now known by many in the scientific world as *neurocardiology*. Loosely defined, neurocardiology is the study of the interaction between heart and brain. We will examine this area and the ideas behind it in chapter 8.

Researchers at HeartMath have used technology to look into these patterns of heart-brain communication, and coined the phrase *heart intelligence* to describe how the heart receives and processes information and sends it to the brain. Laboratories all over the world are now engaged in this area of study.

As these patterns of heart-to-brain communication were better understood, Doc Childre and the team at HeartMath were able to develop very simple and easily learned tools to help people transform stress by changing the underlying physiological and biochemical reactions that take place inside the body quite automatically. One reason why these tools work so well is that the electrical signals from the heart are roughly fifty times stronger than the signals from the brain! The HeartMath work has been fascinating, and people all over the globe have been able to employ these tools to lower stress and increase performance—in the corporate world, schools, all four branches of the military, and especially in health care. You'll get to read some of their stories in the latter half of the book.

It turns out that use of the HeartMath tools also produces a drop in blood pressure in many people who use them. This observation, while not unexpected, has provided doctors with an entirely new approach to the treatment of hypertension. Readers of this book will learn the scientific background of this research, and also learn the tools that have been very effective for so many who use them for lowering stress and blood pressure.

Many people have been able to use the HeartMath tools to avoid the need for medications. Some have been able to lessen the amount of medications taken. Some have gotten off their medicines completely. Just as is the case with pills, there are some for whom the tools won't lower their blood pressure. But there are never any side effects to HeartMath, except living healthier, living better, performing at higher levels, and appreciating life to a much greater extent.

How HeartMath Found Me

My own introduction to HeartMath came in 1997. At the time, I was researching methods of stress reduction for patients with heart disease. Abundant medical literature had been accumulating over the prior decade that clearly demonstrated the link between stress and heart trouble — especially the connection between hypertension and coronary artery disease, which causes heart attacks and more deaths than any other illness in the United States and most other developed countries. The exact mechanisms were not understood, but doctors knew that those who had suffered a heart attack or needed bypass surgery fared much worse and had a much higher chance of having another cardiac problem if stress in their lives was not addressed in some way. There was also strong evidence that relieving stress in these individuals actually reduced the likelihood of future cardiac events (heart attacks, being hospitalized again, needing angioplasty or surgery, or death). There were even data on how many health care dollars could be saved if stress could be lessened in these patients.

So I went on a search to see how patients in cardiac rehabilitation programs were being taught stress reduction, or if they were being taught it at all. I found many different methods being taught in many different ways, but nobody was measuring the amount of stress relief being achieved, because it was not measurable. There was no yardstick for stress, or its interruption.

Most people, whether they went to medical school or not, know that excess stress is harmful. As a cardiologist, I had been trained to modify risk factors for heart disease. I was adept at using medications to lower blood pressure, drop cholesterol levels in the blood, help people to stop smoking, and reduce blood sugar in diabetics. About the only thing I felt I couldn't do was change the parents of my patients (many of whom had already had that idea). My frustration was that stress remained behind the black curtain—no one could measure it, so it was difficult to know how much benefit came to those who were able to lessen it, and by what mechanism.

Then my world changed, quite by accident. A man who worked in the hospital where I was doing all my cardiology work approached me one day with an article in his hand from *Natural Health Magazine* (Thomson 1997). He said, "Hey, you're a heart doctor; what do you know about this Heart-Math stuff?" I told him that I had never heard of it. He handed me the magazine and I told him that I would get back to him the following week at a meeting that both of us would be attending.

I read the article that same day. It was clear by about the fourth paragraph that some very interesting pieces of a long-standing puzzle were coming together. I read about the Institute of HeartMath in Boulder Creek, California, started by Doc Childre, a man vitally interested in our innate responses to stress and the effect of those biological reactions on our health, our performance, our perceptions, and ultimately our well-being. The language in the article captivated me. I decided to contact the Institute.

The man who answered the phone was a British physicist who was part of the HeartMath team. I told him all about my career in academic medicine and cardiology, and that I was fascinated with what his colleagues at the Institute had learned about how the heart signal was so powerful, and how they were able to observe its influence over brain functions, immunity, blood pressure, and many other things related to health. I asked him if I might visit their laboratory. He told me that he thought it would be best, in light of my interest in helping my cardiac patients, for me to take the stress reduction seminar myself. While I was there, he would be happy to introduce me to the research team and arrange for me to spend some time at the lab if that was my desire.

Three weeks later I boarded an airplane, armed with a fistful of articles on something called heart rate variability (HRV). This is the tool that the scientists at HeartMath had used to gain a window into the inner workings of the heart and the nervous system. (We'll spend a lot of time on that subject in this book.)

After the arrival of about twenty other attendees, dinner was served. We were assembled after dinner in the conference room, where thousands of people have learned the HeartMath tools over the years. Dr. Rollin McCraty, the laboratory director, spent about an hour showing us slides that described the fascinating research that had been done there, along with work on HRV that had been accomplished in other laboratories around the world.

Perhaps it was because I am a cardiologist, or perhaps it was just because I am who I am, but I was completely captivated with the beauty and simplicity of their work and their findings. Over the course of the next few days I learned the science and vocabulary of how people communicate with themselves internally during different emotional states and when confronted by various threats, either real or imagined. I learned the physiology of the stress response and why people behave the way they do when under stress, and how it affects their health in the moment and in the long term. Sort of funny for a cardiologist who had been educated at some very prestigious institutions, yet really knew nothing about this! But nobody else knew much about this, either. That's what research is all about—learning new things, and realizing how wrong we all are until the next layer of the onion gets peeled and we see what's underneath.

This research was the foundation of understanding the power of the heart, quite literally. I had been taught that the heart was simply a pump, just as you were. But here I learned how the heart has its own "little brain" composed of thousands of nerve cells that send very influential information to the brain on top of your shoulders. Once this discovery was understood by the HeartMath research team and they began measuring the information the heart was sending, they were able to devise very simple tools that help people break the stress response. As I mentioned earlier, an overactive stress response becomes quite toxic to health, and millions of us are actually dying faster than we need to because of all the negative effects that stress has on so many of our internal systems.

I could see immediately that the tools taught in this program should not just be limited to those who could make the long and winding trip to this incredible place in the coastal redwoods of California, but should be integrated into health care in general. After all, I had started out looking for scientifically documented, measurable, and successful ways of breaking the stress response for heart patients.

I spoke to some of the staff at HeartMath about my idea of integrating their methods into cardiac rehab programs. I told them that hospitals themselves had become very stressful places for many reasons — regulations, chronically ill patients with acute problems, fearful families, and demanding schedules to name just a few (no mention here of unreasonable doctors, you'll note). I therefore also felt we should make these tools available to nurses and other hospital employees so they could better cope with the stresses of their work, and ultimately give better care to their patients.

I can tell you that when I returned home and proposed a pilot program in my own hospital, I was greeted with a look from the president of my hospital that told me he thought I might have ingested a toxic substance while visiting California. Although I persevered, and fought endlessly for the development of this program, it took the curiosity of Diane Ball, a nurse who heard me speak of HeartMath at a national cardiac rehabilitation meeting, to really get the ball rolling. The results in her institution (Delnor Hospital in Aurora, Illinois) have been spectacular, and have been reproduced in other hospitals. The Health Care Division at HeartMath was created in the process. The rest, as they say, is history, and it's being written right now.

I have been delivering lectures on the science of HeartMath and seminars to teach these tools since 1997. It is a real passion for me. I will often teach individual patients these tools in my office, as well. Whether it's to reduce their blood pressure, or to enable them to alleviate stress and its many negative effects for any number of other reasons, the HeartMath program has been what many of my patients have called a "lifesaver."

I invite you to accompany me on a short journey. You'll learn a lot about blood pressure, its effects, and its treatments. Best of all, you'll learn how to use the remarkably easy and effective HeartMath tools to cut stress in all aspects of your life. If we happen to lower your blood pressure in the process, we'll be happier and you'll be healthier. If this sounds a little too good to be true, remember that I'm a doctor, and a heart doctor at that. You have to believe me. It's a rule. Read on.

Chapter 1

What Is Blood Pressure?

Blood pressure is the force of the blood pushing out against the walls of the blood vessels. As blood is pumped out of the heart into the arteries that lead away from it, there is a certain pressure in the system created by this pumping action of the heart.

Measuring Blood Pressure

Blood pressure is measured in a few different ways, but the most common method at the time this book is being written is called *sphygmomanometry* (SFIG-mo-man-AH-muh-tree). It's a big and unwieldy word that refers to inflating a blood pressure cuff on the arm (or leg, in some cases). Air is slowly let out of the cuff while the person taking your blood pressure listens with a stethoscope below the cuff to hear the pulse.

When the person first hears the pulse as the cuff deflates, the pressure is recorded as the *systolic* pressure. It's called that because with each beat, the heart squeezes blood out of the main pumping chamber—the *left ventricle*—into the main blood pipe leaving the heart, called the *aorta*. This contraction of the heart muscle that ejects blood out into the "pipes" of your circulatory system is called *systole* (SIS-toh-lee). So every time the heart beats, the blood that is ejected during systole creates a rise in pressure in the arteries — the branches off the aorta that carry blood away from the heart to all of the organs and muscles of your body. It just so happens that a convenient artery in which to measure your blood pressure is in your arm, but as mentioned above, it can be measured in the leg also, or almost anywhere else in your body if special equipment is used.

Everybody knows that there are two numbers recorded when blood pressure is measured. We talked about the top number above. The bottom number is called the *diastolic* pressure. It reflects the pressure in the arteries when it is at its lowest, right before the heart pumps blood out into the system again. During *diastole* (dye-ASS-toh-lee), the heart is relaxing and filling up with blood. So, blood pressure is recorded as two numbers:

systolic pressure

---

diastolic pressure

A Closed System

The circulatory system is a closed system. This means that there are no valves anywhere in the pipes to let blood out. In addition to the pumping and filling of the heart, pressure is maintained in this closed system by the tension in the walls of the arteries.

Arteries have a layer of muscle in their walls. This muscle layer can contract or relax and have a great impact on the pressure in the overall system. Arteries that supply blood to muscles and organs have the ability to dilate (enlarge) under conditions when more blood is required. For example, if you are running, the muscles in your legs need more oxygenated blood because they're working harder. So the arteries feeding your leg muscles relax and expand in order to deliver the needed fuel to your muscles.

When your arteries dilate, the pressure in the entire circulatory system would drop, except for the fact that your heart is pumping harder and faster to help increase the blood supply to the leg muscles that need it. This boosts pressure instead. In addition, the contraction of those leg muscles helps to squeeze the arteries and veins (veins have the job of bringing blood back to the heart) while you are running, maintaining pressure in the system.

There is a wonderful and incredible balance in the body. If the brain senses a drop in blood pressure, the heart speeds up and also pumps harder. A message is also sent to the arteries to "clamp down," or constrict, and raise the pressure back toward normal. If blood pressure gets too low, you feel faint, because not enough blood is getting to your brain. You turn pale. This is because the arteries in the skin are all contracting at the same time to help raise the pressure and maintain blood flow to the vital organs of the body.

On the other hand, if you get overheated, the arteries in the skin dilate in order to get more of your blood to the surface of the body, so the heat can be radiated out into the atmosphere. A message is also sent to your sweat glands to squeeze water through your skin, so as it evaporates you are cooled down.

The blood pressure is therefore maintained by the constriction and relaxation of the arteries as well as the pumping of the heart. There is an elaborate series of feedback mechanisms in place so that the pressure doesn't drop too low or get too high in a healthy person.

Problems with Blood Pressure

Problems occur in the body when the blood pressure gets too high (hypertension) or too low (hypotension).

What Is Hypertension?

Hypertension is the medical term for high blood pressure. *Hyper* means "too much," and *tension*, of course, means "pressure." That part is easy. What's not easy is figuring out what causes it most of the time. We'll get to that later.

Most people have been told that "normal" blood pressure is 120/80. Every few years, experts in the field meet to review scientific research and the current guidelines on blood pressure in order to update them if necessary. Currently, blood pressure is classified as:

Normal (optimal): less than 120 systolic and less than 80 diastolic

Prehypertension: 120–139 systolic *or* 80–89 diastolic, or both

Stage 1 Hypertension: 140–159 systolic *or* 90–99 diastolic, or both

Stage 2 Hypertension: greater than 160 systolic *or* greater than 100 diastolic, or both (Chobanian et al. 2003)

So, if your systolic pressure is greater than 130, and your diastolic pressure is over 80, you have some degree of hypertension.

Scope of the Problem

Research published in 2004 (Fields et al.) indicates that the number of adults with hypertension in the United States had risen from fifty million to sixty-five million during the previous ten years. Before 2004, we were shocked to learn that one in four adults in America had hypertension. Now it's even more—one-third of adults have it!

Symptoms of Hypertension

The majority of people who develop high blood pressure are completely unaware of it. This means that it is important to check blood pressure periodically because it can be elevated, and often is, with no symptoms at all. In fact, many symptoms that are commonly associated with hypertension—headache, nosebleed, dizziness, and fainting—are seen just as commonly in people with normal blood pressure. Often these symptoms of hypertension are also associated with complications from the disease (see chapter 3).

A Word About Low Blood Pressure

Blood pressure can indeed be too low. If someone has an accident that causes excessive bleeding, the pressure will drop. Certain medications (some of them used to treat high blood pressure) can lower the pressure too far. Various neurological conditions can cause sudden drops in blood pressure, causing fainting in more severe cases.

When blood pressure gets very low, you go into shock. This implies that there isn't enough pressure in the system to adequately push blood through the arteries to the vital organs that keep you alive, like the heart and the brain. It is obviously a life-threatening condition.

Milder drops in blood pressure that don't threaten life are called *hypotension* (*hypo* means "under," or too low). Some people do just fine with blood pressures of 85/50, and doctors treat some people with conditions such as congestive heart failure to reduce their pressures down to these levels. Other people feel terrible when their systolic pressure drops from 150 down to 130. Like everything else in life, everyone is different, and it's not the number that counts; it's how well the person is doing and feeling.

In chapters 2 through 5, we're going to discuss problems related to hypertension and then the drugs and lifestyle changes that help to lower blood pressure.

Feel free to jump directly to chapter 6 and the chapters that follow to get to the heart of the matter and learn the HeartMath tools. You can always come back to the technical sections.

Chapter 2

Causes of High Blood Pressure

This may seem surprising to you, but in the vast majority of cases, doctors have no idea what causes hypertension. They know the predictors that can contribute to it, such as stress, obesity, and diabetes, but this isn't the same as the cause. In medicine, when doctors don't know the cause of something, it's usually referred to as *idiopathic*, meaning "we're idiots when it comes to knowing the cause." When doctors don't know the cause of high blood pressure, a special term is used called *essential hypertension* (also called *primary* hypertension). Unfortunately, essential hypertension is the diagnosis in 90 to 95 percent of people who have high blood pressure. That's unfortunate because it offers no insight into a cause that might be treatable, or even preventable.

The origins of the term "essential" hypertension refer to an outdated idea that a rise in blood pressure was necessary to maintain balance in the human system. It was viewed as an adaptive reaction. Dr. John Hay, writing in the *British Medical Journal* in 1931, opined that doctors shouldn't measure blood pressure because they might feel compelled to lower it.

This notion was very common at the time, and probably contributed to the delay in realizing the dangers of hypertension. It also put a damper on the idea that lowering the pressure might be helpful. Many doctors held this belief well into the late 1940s.

Dr. R. W. Scott, a prominent physician in the middle of the last century, speculated that elevated blood pressure might very well be a natural response, guaranteeing a more normal circulation to the vital organs of the body (hence the term "essential hypertension").

In modern times, even though the exact causes of hypertension remain a mystery most of the time, it's known that there are some conditions that may cause high blood pressure or make it worse. Physicians often screen patients for these conditions when they see the pressure is unusually high, and will dig deeper or refer the patient to a specialist if the patient does not respond to recommended lifestyle changes and/or medication.

Doctors generally make sure that the blood pressure really is high before prescribing medications to bring the pressure down. Some people have "white coat hypertension," which means that their pressure is only high when they are at the doctor's office. While this condition usually needs no treatment, physicians want to make sure this is actually the case through repeated testing. Real hypertension is very common and leads to many other illnesses and complications if not detected and treated in some way to bring the pressure back to the normal or optimal range.

Despite an inability to come up with the exact cause of high blood pressure in the majority of cases, physicians know that there are a number of factors which may predispose individuals to hypertension. Looking at these factors can help reveal better approaches to prevention and treatment.

Genetics

Not many years ago, the medical community felt that researchers would find "the gene" responsible for high blood pressure, just as they've identified certain genetic markers for other diseases. That turned out to be naive, since it seems now that many genes are involved. It is true, though, that hypertension can and does run in certain families. You are more likely to develop high blood pressure if others in your family have had it.

Hypertension in African-Americans

Over the years it has become obvious that high blood pressure acts a little differently in the African-American population. African-Americans have an increased incidence and prevalence of hypertension, and higher complication rates, including death, than whites or other ethnic groups. They also have a higher incidence of kidney damage as a result of high blood pressure, and more patients progress to the point of kidney failure and dialysis.

Much speculation has been offered as to why this might be the case. African ancestors lived in hot, dry climates, which required their bodies to conserve salt (sodium) and water internally. This worked well when their intake of sodium was low, as was the case on the African continent. But as the population migrated and time passed, the diets became much higher in salt. Some researchers think that African-Americans living in cultures with higher salt intake may be more susceptible to "sodium overload." It has been observed, for example, that when the Xhosa people of South Africa migrated to urban areas and increased their sodium intake, they suffered a significant rise in their blood pressures (Sever et al. 1980).

Whatever the reasons, doctors know that hypertension seems like a different disease in African-Americans. A greater effort needs to be made, therefore, to screen this population and treat them aggressively, by any means, in hopes of lessening the dangerous outcomes. It also means that their treatments should be tailored more specifically to aim at getting rid of excess salt and water as a first line of therapy.

Obesity

Obesity is a very strong contributor to hypertension. Being significantly overweight is an epidemic in many countries today. It's an ongoing disease, not a cosmetic problem. It affects you in many ways—not just how you look.

Obesity is a complex disease that is a consequence of taking in more calories than you burn off. It is influenced by many factors, such as family history, race, level of activity, and environment. Portion size is a major contributor to overeating. Fast-food restaurants often give people more calories in one meal than they need in an entire day.

As society progressed from a time when it was necessary to do physical work all day (hunt for food, grow food, and build dwellings) to the modern era, when most work is done from a chair while staring at a computer screen, people simply burned fewer calories. All of the modern conveniences have left people melting into the couch.

Obesity contributes to other diseases as well. Type 2 diabetes was usually seen in middle age as a direct consequence of obesity. Now it's showing up in children as they get fatter. Type 2 diabetes contributes to coronary artery disease, eye disease, and many other conditions, including premature death.

Obesity is also a strong risk factor for the development of high cholesterol and heart disease. *Sleep apnea*, a disease of disordered breathing during sleep causing many other medical complications, is also predominantly a disease of the overweight.

So obesity creates many problems, not the least of which is hypertension. The bottom line here is this: Weight gain is associated with higher blood pressure, which can contribute to many other diseases.

Lack of Physical Activity

Modern technology allows you to accomplish much more while physically doing much less. When was the last time you changed the channel on your TV set by getting up and walking across the room?

People who engage in regular, sustained physical activity have lower blood pressures. They also have less obesity, less heart trouble, and less depression. Many people feel that they must engage in strenuous activity like running or weight lifting to lower their risk of these diseases. While more vigorous exercise can provide other benefits, simply walking for thirty to forty minutes a day has been shown to be sufficient for lowering disease risk.

Regular exercise, especially *aerobic* exercise (sustained exercise that raises the heart rate but doesn't put sudden strain on your system like heavy weight lifting), has many benefits beyond lowering blood pressure. It can:

- Strengthen the heart and cardiovascular system

- Help your muscles to utilize the oxygen delivered by the blood more efficiently
- Improve energy levels and endurance
- Improve muscle strength
- Strengthen bones
- Increase flexibility and balance
- Reduce body fat
- Help to reduce tension, stress, and depression
- Improve sleep
- Increase self-esteem

Excess Salt in the Diet

Too much salt in the diet can be harmful. The chemical name for salt is sodium chloride. Nutrition labels on foods now list how much sodium is contained in a serving of whatever is in the box, can, or bottle. Sodium is present in high amounts in certain types of foods. Ketchup and pickles are great examples of high-sodium foods. Many canned soups and most snack-food items (potato chips, corn chips, and the like) are very high in salt also. Any type of meat that has preservatives to prolong its shelf life, such as sausage, hot dogs, or bacon, will contain high levels of sodium.

One of the problems with salt intake is that some people seem to be more sensitive to salt than others, meaning that they are more likely to develop hypertension in response to excess sodium in their diet. There is no way to predict who might be salt sensitive. There has been extensive research over many years on salt and its potential contribution to high blood pressure. Evidence for this causative role includes the following:

- In large populations, the prevalence of hypertension rises with the levels of sodium intake.

- Most groups with very low sodium intake have no hypertension. When higher levels of salt are introduced, hypertension develops.

- Certain animals seem predisposed to high blood pressure when fed high-sodium diets.

- Despite the fact that less than half of people are salt sensitive, dietary salt restriction will lower blood pressure in most people.

Age

As you get older, you'll naturally lose "stretch" in many of your tissues. Your blood vessels are no exception. *Elasticity* is the word that describes how stretchable something is. As you age, the elasticity in your arteries decreases. This means that when the heart is pumping blood into the arteries, the pressure will rise if the arteries have lost some of their ability to expand. Picture arteries made of soft rubber. Each time the heart squeezes, it ejects blood into the pipes to keep it circulating around the system. As the pipes grow stiffer over time, the pressure in the system will go up if the volume of blood being pumped remains the same. This is sometimes referred to as "hardening of the arteries." This term is also used to describe the buildup of plaque on the inside of the arteries, especially the heart. But you get the idea — as the pipes lose their ability to stretch over the years, they don't absorb the shock of the pulse as well as they used to. Rigid pipes make for higher pressure.

People at Increased Risk for Development of Hypertension

You have an increased risk of having hypertension if you:

- are over the age of thirty-five

- are overweight

- eat foods that are high in salt or fat, or both

- are not active

- smoke

- drink excess alcohol (more than two drinks per day)

- have family members who have high blood pressure

- are African-American

- are pregnant

- take oral contraceptives (birth control pills)

- are under stress

We will spend a great deal of time on the last topic on the list, but first let's look at some of the medical conditions that can cause high blood pressure.

Secondary Hypertension

Secondary hypertension is the name given to high blood pressure that is known to be caused by something else. Only about 5 percent of high blood pressure falls in this category. Many other diseases can elevate blood pressure by a number of mechanisms.

The Kidneys

The kidneys are frequently the cause of hypertension for many reasons. This is because the kidneys help to regulate blood pressure. As blood is pumped out of the heart into the main artery, the aorta, it travels throughout the body. The aorta gives off many arteries that feed all of the organs, muscles, and other structures. When blood goes through the kidneys, it passes through the renal (kidney) arteries. The kidneys are very complex filtering machines that filter out toxins that will then leave the body via the urine.

Blood passes from the aorta through the renal artery and into the kidney itself, where it is pushed through a fine mesh of very small blood vessels that act like a sieve. After going through this filter, the blood travels through a loop of blood vessels that control salt and water balance. This allows water to be reabsorbed back into your circulation to keep everything in balance. Ultimately, toxins and whatever salt and water you don't need pass from the kidneys down pipes called *ureters* into the bladder, which you empty periodically when the urge hits you. Now things get a little more complicated. If you were to design a monitoring system to keep track of blood pressure (too low—just right—too high), the kidney might not be such a bad place to put this monitor. After all, the blood has to circulate through the kidneys at the proper pressure to filter out toxins and balance salt and water.

If the kidney sees low pressure, it might get nervous that not enough pushing pressure is present to adequately filter out the bad stuff. This could be because the blood pressure actually is low, or because there may be a partial blockage of the renal artery with cholesterol, just as can happen in the heart. Another condition related to this is called *fibromuscular dysplasia.* This is always considered when a young woman develops hypertension because as rare as this problem is, it is almost never seen in men or older women. For some reason, scar tissue forms in the mouth of the renal artery, thus decreasing blood flow to the kidney. Luckily, this is easily treated in most cases with angioplasty, just like doctors treat partially blocked arteries in the heart. Angioplasty is performed by placing a balloon into an artery under X-ray guidance and blowing it up to open the channel for better blood flow.

Regardless of the cause, when the kidney "sees," or thinks it sees, low pressure, it produces a hormone called *renin* (REE-nin). This hormone is spilled from the kidney into the circulation and acts on another chemical, which then acts on another, and in the long run the message goes to the arteries in the body to squeeze down, thus raising the overall pressure in the system. This phenomenon of contracting arteries in the body is known as *vasoconstriction* (*vaso* means "blood vessel"). The arteries have muscles in their walls for exactly this reason.

Imagine you lived thousands of years ago, and while you were walking through the jungle, you encountered a tiger that was inconsiderate enough to nip your leg. You would lose a lot of blood, and, of course, your blood pressure would drop. Your kidneys would sense this drop in filtering pressure and pour the hormone renin into your bloodstream. This would start a long chain reaction that would eventually cause your blood vessels to constrict, thus raising the pressure and keeping you alive. If your blood pressure drops too low, your brain stops working and your heart stops beating. This is considered to be disadvantageous in most circles.

Another consequence of renin production by the kidneys is the triggering of the production and release of other hormones and chemicals from the *adrenal glands*, which sit on top of the kidneys. These substances not only contribute to the constriction of the arteries, but also pass through the kidneys and cause them to reabsorb salt and water back into the circulatory system, thus helping to raise blood pressure by maintaining the fluid volume in your blood vessels.

One could imagine that many things might go wrong in this complicated organ called the kidney. (And you thought its only job on earth was to make urine and wake you up in the middle of the night!) Many diseases, including hypertension itself, can create damage to the kidney. Tumors, infection, diabetes, autoimmune diseases (lupus, for example) or kidney stones can also cause kidney problems resulting in higher blood pressure. As mentioned above, buildup of cholesterol in the renal artery can create a partial blockage and thereby decrease blood flow into the kidney, fooling it into thinking the blood pressure in the entire system is low, triggering renin production and raising pressure.

The Adrenal Glands

We just mentioned the adrenal glands in the last section. One of their jobs is to respond to signals originating in the kidney, but sometimes they act on their own.

Each adrenal (*ad* means "on top of"; *renal* means "kidney") gland looks like a little triangular hat sitting atop the kidney below it. It is made up of two parts: the middle core, known as the *medulla*, and the outer layer, known as the *cortex* (cover). The medulla makes *adrenaline* (whoa — what a coincidence — adrenaline being made in the adrenal gland!). It also makes and stores a couple of other closely related compounds, which quickly and markedly raise blood pressure in a crisis situation.

The outer cortex of each adrenal gland makes a hormone called *aldosterone* (al-DOSS-ter-ohn). Aldosterone is a very powerful compound that travels (not very far) by way of the blood to the kidney, where it tells the kidney to reabsorb sodium (salt) before it goes out in the urine. Since everything in the body must remain in balance, water is reabsorbed along with the sodium.

All of this filtering, excreting, and reabsorbing goes along for years without a hitch to make sure you get rid of toxins and things you don't need, while saving things that you do need. But problems can occur, causing increased sodium and water reabsorption and retention, and you get bloated. This bloating usually occurs inside your blood vessels. In other words, your blood has more liquid in it, and that pushes against the inside of your blood vessels, raising your blood pressure.

As discussed earlier, only about 5 to 10 percent of high blood pressure has a known cause (so it's called secondary hypertension, remember?). But of all the causes for hypertension, these disorders in the adrenal gland are probably the most common. And doctors are finding that a number of cases that were diagnosed as essential hypertension were really caused by overactive adrenal gland tissue. It can be sort of tricky to ferret out this problem and make the diagnosis, so physicians have missed it in some people.

Other Problems

We've seen how the kidney makes its own hormone, renin, that raises blood pressure when it senses that the blood flow lacks proper force. It's a built-in system to prevent you from dying of too little blood pressure (also called "shock"). As stated earlier, the kidney can be fooled by a partial blockage in the renal artery that feeds it, either by cholesterol or by scar tissue. It can also be affected by a myriad of hormones produced in other glands around the body. We spent some time talking about the adrenal glands, both when they function normally and when they produce too much of one substance or another that elevate blood pressure, sometimes rather wildly.

Nerve signals and hormones from the brain serve as messengers to raise blood pressure often through many steps. Pain or cold temperatures can do this, too. Fortunately, these are only temporary conditions in most cases.

So while most hypertension is primary, or essential—without a known cause—a few cases are secondary to other illnesses or conditions. When a doctor diagnoses high blood pressure, he or she will decide how diligently to look for the known causes, since they are only present about 5 to 10 percent of the time. Certain basic screening tests are usually ordered, and treatment recommended when necessary. But to look for all sorts of rare causes in every patient is not cost-effective, given that high blood pressure is so common and the secondary causes are so rare. Physicians will often think about these other causes when there's something unusual, like young age, certain specific signs or symptoms, or a sudden rise in blood pressure when it was normal or under good control in the past.

Keep your eyes on the adrenal glands—they're going to turn up again when we discuss how stress affects people in many more ways than just elevating blood pressure.

Chapter 3

Dangers of High Blood Pressure: Why Should You Treat It?

The problem with high blood pressure is that most people can't feel it. That means that a person could have elevated blood pressure for a long period of time and be completely unaware of it. Doctors learned quite a bit about the consequences of hypertension by leaving it alone for years. Unfortunately, they got a very good lesson about what goes wrong when blood pressure stays high. There are a number of organs and structures that are the "targets" of chronically elevated blood pressure. This chapter deals with target organ damage, which you should be aware of.

The Heart

The heart is known as the most important organ in the body for obvious reasons—it pumps blood all through the body to deliver oxygen and other nutrients for proper functioning.

Some would argue that the brain is more important than the heart, since it doesn't make much sense to be alive if your heart is pumping away and you cannot function. But if the heart goes, everything goes.

Many things can go wrong with the heart over time, but hypertension exerts a particularly harmful influence on it. Heart disease is the number-one killer of people in most countries. But what do we mean by *heart disease*?

Coronary Artery Disease (CAD)

The most common form of heart disease is *coronary artery disease*. The coronary arteries are the ones that sit on the surface of the heart, sending branches down into the heart muscle to nourish it with fresh oxygen. The term *coronary* means "like a crown" — the arteries encircle the heart on its surface much like a crown might.

The main problem with arteries is that they get clogged. This occurs when there is inflammation of the artery wall and scar tissue forms. Cholesterol is a big contributor to the inflammation, and it becomes part of the scar tissue in the artery wall. These cholesterol deposits are called *plaques*.

Hypertension also contributes to the inflammation and scar tissue formation by exerting a greater force against the inside of the artery wall. This concept is called *shear force*, since the column of blood coursing through the blood vessels at a higher pressure can cause small tears in the lining, resulting in damage and inflammation. Nicotine from cigarettes causes a chemical inflammation of the artery wall. Therefore, a smoker with high cholesterol and high blood pressure will have a very high likelihood of getting coronary artery disease. It is important to control blood pressure because the higher it is, the faster plaque develops.

Heart Attack

The dangerous and often deadly consequence of CAD is *heart attack.* The medical term for heart attack is *myocardial infarction* (*myo* means "heart;" *cardial* means "muscle;" *infarction* means "tissue death"). Heart attack is a very specific term; it means the sudden blockage of blood flow to the heart muscle, resulting in the death of a segment of this muscle. Heart attack doesn't mean dropping over, although some people do drop over. In fact, about half of the people who die of a heart attack do so before reaching a hospital.

Contrary to what you might think, heart attack doesn't happen because more and more cholesterol builds up on the inside of a coronary artery like rings on a tree. Instead, one of the plaques actually ruptures. Why this happens all of a sudden is the subject of a great deal of medical research.

Congestive Heart Failure (CHF)

This is a term with a rather nasty sound to it. *Heart failure* makes it sound like a person is making a beeline for the inside of a pine box. But people with this diagnosis can actually live for a very long time, thanks to many advances in medicine over the past fifty years or so.

Heart failure is really a constellation of problems rather than a disease. It means that the heart is not functioning properly, so that blood is not being pumped around the body efficiently. The end result is that your tissues are not receiving adequate blood supply to meet their needs. People with heart failure frequently suffer from fatigue. They also tire easily when exerting themselves, because decreased pumping action from the heart does not deliver enough blood to the leg muscles during walking or other exercise.

But the most common reason for the heart not to be pumping well enough to meet the body's needs is coronary artery disease. People who have had one or more heart attacks lose heart muscle in the process. The more heart muscle that is lost, the weaker the pump. This can happen with one big heart attack, or a number of smaller ones over time.

How High Blood Pressure Causes Heart Failure

As blood pressure rises, it provides higher and higher resistance to the blood flowing out of the heart into the aorta. The higher the resistance in the "pipes," the harder the pump has to squeeze to get the blood out into the system to feed the organs and muscles. At first, the heart muscle thickens as it pumps minute after minute, hour after hour, against this resistance. Think of your biceps muscle on your upper arm as you hold a five-pound weight in your hand, bending your elbow to lift this weight an average of seventy-two times a minute—forever. At first your muscle gets larger (you might even get a date!), but eventually your arm will tire and become weaker, unable to lift the weight and eventually unable to flex your elbow even without the weight in your hand.

The same is true for the heart. So if high blood pressure goes undetected or untreated for a long time, your heart muscle gets progressively weaker. It doesn't actually fail, at least not until the bitter end, but it fails to meet the needs of the tissues that have a lot of work to do.

What about the *congestive* part? As the heart weakens, blood, and hence pressure, backs up in the system. The lungs can't empty blood into the heart as well because of this pressure backup, and therefore become *congested* with blood themselves. This causes some of the water in the blood to squeeze through the very thin walls of the blood vessels and into the air sacs of the lungs. That makes it harder to breathe, because oxygen can't pass through the air sacs into the blood vessels when the air sacs are flooded with water. The pressure continues to back up into the right side of the heart, which has the job of pumping blood into the lungs. Then blood has trouble getting back into the heart from the body.

Eventually this backup causes *edema*, or swelling, in the rest of the body, especially the ankles. When the heart can't pump adequately, people get *fatigued* (there is inadequate blood supply to muscles), and develop shortness of breath when they try to exert themselves. As CHF gets worse, these symptoms not only occur during times of exertion, but also with less and less activity, and finally even while a person is at rest.

Hypertension was the most common cause of congestive heart failure up until the middle of the last century. Because of this, there was finally a push to treat blood pressure and return it to normal levels. More aggressive therapy for high blood pressure has dropped it into second place as a cause of CHF, but far too many people still suffer from this syndrome.

The Brain

The brain is very sensitive to high blood pressure, both acutely (moment to moment) and chronically (over the long term).

Stroke

Stroke is very much like a heart attack in that tissue dies as a result of interrupted blood flow. In this case, it's brain tissue, not heart muscle. Stroke has therefore been called by some a "brain attack."

The Two Mechanisms of Stroke

Stroke, known in medicine as a *cerebrovascular accident*, or CVA, can occur for two reasons. The most common reason is that a little chunk of cholesterol plaque, just like that which is present in the coronary arteries of the heart, breaks loose from a blood vessel supplying the brain and travels up into smaller and smaller vessels, finally getting stuck when the size of the chunk is bigger than the vessel it is traveling in. This cuts off blood flow to a segment of the brain. The resultant loss of function is related to where in the brain this floating plug, or *embolus*, ends up. It may cause damage in the area that controls speech. It may create problems in motor areas of the brain, causing loss of function of an arm, or a leg, or both. Facial drooping on one side may be the result of loss of function in the muscles of facial expression.

Blood clots also *embolize* (break off and travel elsewhere). Some blood clots may form in the heart, while others originate elsewhere and pass through the heart, eventually moving into a vessel in the brain. Whether it's a blood clot or a bit of cholesterol debris, the floating material eventually gets to a point in the brain circulation where it blocks flow and tissue dies. These strokes, known as *embolic* strokes, regardless of what the embolic material is, are by far the most common type, accounting for about 85 percent of all strokes.

The other type of stroke is caused by rupture of one of the blood vessels in the brain. The most common reason for this, as you might guess, is high blood pressure. When pressure gets too high one of these vessels may burst, causing bleeding or *hemorrhage* in the brain. *Hemorrhagic* stroke is usually more serious and harder to recover from than embolic stroke. *Aneurysm*, or weakening in the wall of the arteries (in the brain in this case), can be the source of hemorrhagic stroke. An aneurysm looks a little like a bulge on the inner tube of a tire. This segment of the artery wall is thinner and weaker, and can rupture even when the blood pressure is normal. But aneurysms are far more likely to burst and cause a stroke if blood pressure is high.

Dementia

Dementia is a term used to describe decreased cognitive mental function. It is an abnormal process. Although all of us have a certain decline in brain function as we get older, many people are quite sharp well into their nineties or even after age one hundred.

Probably the best-known type of dementia is *Alzheimer's disease*. However, this type is not associated with hypertension. Midlife blood pressure elevations are predictors of other changes in the brain that lead to cognitive impairment and decline, and the risk for the development of dementia can be significantly reduced by normalizing the blood pressure (Hershey 2003).

Hypertensive Encephalopathy

The term *hypertensive encephalopathy* (en-SEF-uh-LAH-path-ee) describes a syndrome of severe hypertension accompanied by brain dysfunction and neurologic impairment. Complete resolution of this dangerous and frightening problem can be achieved if the blood pressure is quickly lowered, usually with intravenous medication in an intensive care environment (Heistad, Lawton, and Talman 2003).

Kidney Disease

It is difficult to separate the cart and the horse when it comes to hypertension and kidney disease, because hypertension both contributes to and accelerates kidney disease and is also a consequence of kidney disease. As kidney function deteriorates, doctors use the term *renal insufficiency*. When kidney function is extremely poor, and eventually absent, it's called *renal failure*. At this point, the patient will die in the course of a couple of weeks if he or she does not undergo *kidney dialysis*, a complicated but routine procedure whereby the blood is withdrawn from a vein, sent through a series of external filters to remove toxins and water, and returned to the circulation. People can live for years while undergoing dialysis, although their quality of life is usually significantly diminished. The other option for a patient with end-stage kidney disease is to undergo a kidney transplant operation.

Hypertension is the most important risk factor for progressive loss of kidney function. People with normal blood pressure and kidney disease usually develop high blood pressure as their kidney function deteriorates, creating a vicious cycle of worsening kidney function and ever-rising blood pressure, ending often in renal failure (Anderson 2003).

Peripheral Arterial Disease (PAD)

Peripheral arterial disease refers to changes in the aorta and its branches, the arteries. We have already discussed *renal artery disease*, in which cholesterol buildup in the renal arteries decreases blood flow into the kidneys and "tricks" the kidneys into thinking the blood pressure is too low. This triggers the release of the kidney hormone renin, which then sets the chain reaction in motion that ends with salt and water reabsorption in the kidney and squeezing of the arteries, thus raising the blood pressure.

Other blood vessels including the aorta itself can be victimized by hypertension. Aortic aneurysms can form along any part of this main blood vessel, or one of its branches. An aneurysm, as discussed earlier in this chapter, is a weakened and expanded segment of artery, much like that seen in an inner tube of a tire before a blowout. As higher blood pressure pounds against the lining of the aorta or any other artery, it can cause a rupture, most often leading to rapid death. Sometimes the force of blood under high pressure will rip the lining of the aorta. This is called *aortic dissection*, or a *dissecting aneurysm* if it occurs in one of the enlarged areas. This can be catastrophic, since rupture can occur if pressure is not lowered. Quite often, urgent surgery is required to repair the aorta. Also quite often, there isn't time.

When cholesterol narrows the *carotid* (cuh-RAH-tidd) arteries that go north from the aorta up to the brain, stroke is a potential problem. When the arteries that go down into the legs are narrowed by this process, known as *atherosclerosis*, people may develop pain in their calf muscles when they walk. The medical name for this is *claudication*, and it is relieved by stopping for a short time. In severe cases, the toes and feet, being the farthest things downstream, lose their blood supply and turn black, a condition known as *gangrene*. Amputation is required.

Hypertension is a very important culprit in all of these problems. When it is combined with diabetes and smoking, the likelihood of developing peripheral arterial disease is much higher.

The Eyes

When you visit your doctor and she places an ophthalmo-scope against her eye to look into yours, she is looking for signs of hypertension, among other things. The eye is the only human organ where the blood vessels can be directly visualized. A number of changes can occur in the arteries, the veins, and the *optic nerve* that connect to the eye, and the *retina*, where vision is detected on the back surface of the eyeball. These changes are graded in terms of severity, and give the physician valuable information about the duration and extent of hypertension. High blood pressure accelerates eye problems caused by diabetes. Treatment for severe diabetic eye complications is more successful when blood pressure is normal.

So now that you've been to medical school (we left out gynecology, orthopedics, and a few other topics), you've seen how far-reaching the effects of high blood pressure are. This is why it is so important to know what your blood pressure is, and to treat it—one way or another—to return it to the normal range and avoid the complications you've been reading about. In the next chapter, we'll review the options for treatment.

Chapter 4

Drug Treatment of Hypertension

When it finally became clear that hypertension was a significant health problem with many negative consequences, the medical community began treating it with drugs earlier and more aggressively. As time has gone by, more physicians have kept a closer eye on their patients with high blood pressure, rather than taking a "wait and see" approach. As different drugs and drug classes were developed, it was noted that many people required more than one drug, a scenario that we'll discuss after talking a bit about the various classes of pharmacologic agents that have been employed.

It wasn't until the 1940s and '50s that big changes in the treatment of hypertension took place, partly due to the fact that President Franklin Delano Roosevelt eventually died of a stroke, but also suffered from congestive heart failure and kidney failure—all complications of his long-standing hypertension (Bruenn 1970). Although many drugs were tried in the early days of treatment, compounds began to be developed in the 1950s through the 1970s that evolved into the newer drug classes currently in use. In the 1980s and '90s a couple more families of medications hit the scene.

Today there are four basic classes of antihypertensive medications used in the treatment of high blood pressure. Occasionally doctors will have to pull out one of the older drugs for a patient who is *refractory*, or not well controlled on the newer agents. We'll concentrate here on the treatments that are commonly used and usually quite effective if the doctor and the patient are willing to persevere and deal with the "art" of medicine, often known as "trial and error." You may have heard of some of the treatments we'll describe in this chapter. Understanding them in greater detail can be helpful in treating high blood pressure.

We will discuss the classes of drugs below, and you can find examples of these medications in the appendix at the back of this book.

Diuretics

Diuretics are drugs that cause the kidney to put out more water. Getting rid of more urine is known in the medical business as *diuresis*, so diuretics are compounds that make people visit the restroom more frequently.

The diuretics were the first of the modern drugs for blood pressure, and were developed in the 1950s. The way they work is to cause more sodium to be excreted into the urine. Remember that water follows salt. The body's balancing mechanisms ensure that water goes out, too.

The most commonly used drug in this category is *hydro-chlorothiazide*, more easily referred to by both doctors and patients as HCTZ. Others are listed in the appendix.

Some people are particularly sensitive to the actions of diuretics. African-Americans, the elderly, diabetics, as well as people with "metabolic syndrome" (obesity, lipid disorders, hypertension, early or established diabetes, and early vascular disease) respond quite well to these drugs (Papademitriou, Sica, and Izzo 2003). People with salt sensitivity are also good candidates for this class of medication.

Side Effects of Diuretics

If the main action of this category of antihypertensives is to rid the patient of water, then an obvious consequence of taking them might be volume (fluid) depletion. This is unusual, especially at a low dose.

When you excrete sodium and water, you also get rid of potassium, another "salt" in your system. Some patients who either require a higher dose of a diuretic or are very sensitive to it can deplete their potassium stores and may require a potassium supplement.

Years ago it was commonly thought that abnormalities in blood lipids (cholesterol, triglycerides) may develop in some patients, along with elevations in blood sugar. At current doses, both of these things are unlikely, but should be mentioned.

Elevations of uric acid, with the resultant development of gout, can occur, although this is uncommon. Magnesium, another salt in the blood, can also drop, which can interact with the low potassium problem and contribute to rhythm disturbances in the heart.

Beta-Blockers

The *beta-blocker* drugs have been around since the 1970s. The Greek letter β is the symbol for beta, so doctors use it frequently when referring to these drugs: β blockers. These drugs decrease the force of contraction of the heart. Recall that with each squeeze of the heart (systole), blood is ejected into the aorta and eventually into all the branching arteries. Arteries possess the quality of elasticity, and therefore stretch a little with each beat of the heart. Beta-blockers, by reducing the force of the heart's contraction, lower the pressure transmitted into the blood vessels. Beta-blockers also reduce heart rate, so it is common for people taking them to notice a slower pulse. In fact, they are often used to slow the heart rate in people who suffer from rhythm disorders characterized by rapid heartbeats.

There are a number of other ways by which beta-blocker drugs may lower blood pressure. Some of them lower resistance in the walls of blood vessels, causing them to dilate, and thus pressure falls. They also blunt some of the signals coming out of the brain and central nervous system. In addition to their use in hypertension, they have widespread application in the treatment of a myriad or different heart conditions. See the appendix for a list of commonly used beta-blockers.

Side Effects of Beta-Blockers

This is a category of medication that might cause trouble in certain types of patients. For example, people who have a history of asthma should not take beta-blockers, because these drugs can trigger asthma. Most people with a condition called *chronic obstructive pulmonary disease*, most commonly known as *emphysema*, should also avoid them. Some disturbances of heart rhythm that can cause slowing of the heart rate can be made markedly worse if these drugs are given to patients with these conditions. As a matter of fact, that's how doctors have learned that some people have these rhythm problems. It is not uncommon for elderly patients to have slower heart rates due to aging and scarring of the electrical conduction system in the heart (the built-in pace-maker and the "wiring" related to it). Oftentimes a slow heartbeat isn't even noticed by a patient, but when beta-blocker drugs are used to treat high blood pressure, the medication may slow the heart rate even further, and symp-toms ranging from mild fatigue to dizziness or fainting spells can occur. Beta-blockers should also be used with extreme caution in diabetic patients taking insulin, since they can mask the symptoms of low blood sugar, or *hypoglycemia*. Although it was commonly believed in the past that beta-blockers may have caused or worsened depression, most psychiatrists no longer believe this to be true.

Angiotensin Converting Enzyme Inhibitors and Angiotensin Receptor Blockers

Back in chapter 2 we talked about causes of high blood pressure. You may recall that the kidney, when it sees (or thinks it sees) low blood pressure, makes a hormone called renin, which triggers a series of reactions that result in higher pressure.

There's an enzyme we need to talk about called *angio-tensin converting enzyme*. Since that's such a long name, let's just call it ACE. In general, enzymes are chemicals found all over the body that help certain reactions take place, sort of like little biochemical helpers.

When renin is released by the kidney, it acts on another substance that is floating around in your bloodstream that was manufactured in the liver. The result is a chemical called *angiotensin* I. ACE converts angiotensin I to *angiotensin II*, a very powerful substance that has the job of constricting blood vessels and raising blood pressure. Remember that this is all part of the great scheme to keep your blood pressure up if it's falling because a tiger bit your leg off and you're bleeding.

All the cells in the body have receptors on them in order to receive chemical messages that are being sent around the body in the blood. Because our bodies are made up of specialized organs and structures that have specific tasks, the receptors on the surfaces of these cells are specialized, too. It makes no sense for your liver to be receiving messages that are aimed at the kidney, or for the special brain cells that tell you what flavor you just tasted to be receiving messages about how much to squeeze on your arteries to raise your blood pressure. So groups of cells with specific jobs have very specific receptors on them.

The muscle layer in the walls of your arteries has receptors for this powerful angiotensin II stuff. When it is circulating in the blood, it lands on these receptors and causes contraction of the muscles, resulting in constriction in the arteries, and thus higher blood pressure.

So if somebody wanted to figure out a way to lower blood pressure, he or she might look at this chain reaction that ends in angiotensin II sitting on the receptors in the walls of your arteries and see that by blocking the converting enzyme that changes angiotensin I into angiotensin II, you might just get the blood pressure to come down. Brilliant!

This trick actually works, and works rather well. But ACE inhibitors have a funny habit of causing an annoying, dry cough in about 15 or 20 percent of the people taking them. For years, people had to simply "live with it" or stop taking the medicine. Then somebody got another bright idea, and that was to make a drug that interfered with the angiotensin II receptors right on the artery walls themselves. Drugs were designed to do just that, and oddly enough they were named *angiotensin receptor blockers* (ARBs). All the good stuff (lower blood pressure) resulted, without the cough seen when ACE was inhibited. Because the ACE inhibitors and angiotensin receptor blockers work in the same general way by not letting the artery walls constrict, we lump them together in one category.

Side Effects of ACE Inhibitors

As mentioned, a dry, nonproductive cough is seen in 15 to 20 percent of people who take ACE inhibitors. This is not seen with ARBs, and that's exactly why they were invented. Deterioration of kidney function, determined by a blood test, must be looked for in patients starting these drugs. A significant rise in the potassium level in the blood can occur and must be evaluated shortly after starting these drugs. ACE inhibitors have a particularly worrisome side effect, which would be characterized as an "allergic reaction," that only occurs in 1 percent of patients taking them. It consists of severe swelling of the lips, mouth, and tongue, and can cause blockage of the airway. This is called *angioneurotic edema*, and is a medical emergency requiring immediate attention. This can also happen with the ARB drugs.

Calcium Channel Blockers

This is a mixed group of drugs that has been quite effective at lowering blood pressure since the 1980s. All of the drugs in this class work on the principle that when calcium enters into a muscle cell, it gets involved in the process of contraction of the muscle. All arteries have a middle layer of muscle, so blocking the entry of calcium into these muscle cells— through the *calcium channels*—will cut down on the muscular constriction in these arteries. The result: lower blood pressure. See the appendix for a table of calcium channel blockers.

Side Effects of Calcium Channel Blockers

Nifedipine and the related drugs in the top part of the table in the appendix can cause ankle swelling (edema). This is just because they are doing a good job of dilating the arteries. As a result, blood pools in the ankles because people spend most of their waking hours in the upright position. It's simply a matter of gravity. Because these drugs are such good artery relaxers, people can also experience flushing and/or a more rapid heartbeat (the heart's normal response to a drop in blood pressure). Verapamil can slow the heart excessively in some susceptible patients, a problem seen much less often with diltiazem.

Other Types of Drugs Used to Treat Hypertension

The four major categories above are the most commonly used drugs in the treatment of high blood pressure. There are other categories of drugs that may be necessary in specific patients with special situations or in patients for whom no combination of the above medications will bring the pressure down. Lists of these medications can be found in the appendix.

Aldosterone Blockers

We reviewed the physiology of aldosterone in chapter 2. Aldosterone is made in the adrenal gland and travels to the kidney to save sodium (salt) and water. It also acts as a constrictor of blood vessels. Blocking aldosterone may lower blood pressure by both mechanisms. These drugs are most often used in conjunction with other drugs, or may be used alone. High potassium is the most common side effect.

Alpha Blockers

If there was a *beta*, there has to be an *alpha*, right? Alpha refers to the constrictive effect of norepinephrine (noradrenaline) on blood vessels. Alpha blockers interfere with this. They are also used for other conditions like frequent nighttime urination in men with enlarged prostate glands.

Sympatholytic Drugs

These are older drugs with numerous side effects, and therefore are rarely used. *Sympatholytic* refers to decreasing the outpouring of nervous system hormones (*sympatho* means "sympathetic," or your fight-or-flight chemistry; *lytic* means "to cut").

Direct Vasodilators

Vasodilator medicines dilate the blood vessels. These meds act directly on the arteries. They are used only in special situations.

An Important Comment on Drugs

Sadly, the fact is that most people will not have their hypertension controlled with only one drug. Most high blood pressure is treated by primary care doctors (family practitioners or internists). Specialists are called in when blood pressure control has not been achieved, or if there are special problems with diagnosis or treatment. By the time this happens, patients may be taking three or four medications for blood pressure alone.

When blood pressure isn't controlled by a low dose of one drug, doctors often will add a second (or third, or fourth) medicine to the mix. This is because as higher doses of any one medication are taken, there is a greater chance for side effects to develop. In addition, there are often multiple and related problems contributing to increased blood pressure. So it's common to see a diuretic combined with any of the other classes of hypertensive drugs. To make it simpler for the patients, some companies have developed combinations of these medications: ACE inhibitor with diuretic, ACE inhibitor with calcium channel blocker, alpha blocker combined with beta-blocker, and so forth.

Here's a general statement that will apply to every drug or other treatment modality in this book:

Just because scientific studies have shown that certain groups of people will respond better (or worse) than others to a particular drug or other intervention, there is no guarantee, or even assumption, that an individual person in that group will respond in the same way.

For most people, this is just plain common sense, but human beings are very complex creatures (have you noticed?). Genetic makeup, lifestyle, age, and other behaviors and conditions all come together to create individuals who may or may not conform to the textbooks on who is supposed to get better on what drug or with what treatment.

Because people can vary so much in how they respond to medications, this often becomes a journey with the doctor, the patient, and perhaps others such as nurses, dieticians, and family members. It's an exploration that always involves trial and error. It requires a relationship of trust, education, and commitment so that the proper outcome is achieved and harm avoided.

If a physician says, "Take this once a day and see me in two weeks," with no other explanation, or if the patient fails to report that he or she developed a rash on the prescribed drug and stopped taking it (no wonder the pressure is still up), the goals of treatment will not be met and the relationship between all involved parties will not be optimal.

No doctor wants to give a patient a drug that will cause a side effect. Doctors sometimes wonder why a patient will go home with a prescription, look it up on the Internet or hear a high-speed verbal warning at the end of a TV ad, and call back saying, "I'm not taking this drug—it can cause impotence" (or hair loss, or heart rhythm abnormalities). The odds of these things happening, of course, are very low. It's usually a matter of not quite enough explanation by the physician or nurse of potential side effects and the likelihood of them occurring. But no doctor can list all of the possible problems, just as no patient should assume a physician would give him or her a drug that would be likely to cause harm.

The purpose of this book is to help you understand your blood pressure and describe some of the treatments that may help you. Now that we've explored the drugs that are used, we'll look into the many ways in which you can help yourself. It's unlikely that there's any doctor who wouldn't jump for joy to have a patient who could avoid the use of medication entirely—really.

Chapter 5

Lifestyle Changes That Help Lower Blood Pressure

For years the medical community has focused on the drug treatment of hypertension. Many people, however, want to play an active role in their own health. They may wish to avoid prescription medications altogether, or they may feel that even if medicines are needed, they would like to do whatever they can themselves to help. There are a number of ways in which you can make a big difference in lowering your blood pressure.

Diet

We discussed in chapter 2 the fact that salt is an important contributor to hypertension. Some people are "salt sensitive," meaning that they have a significant rise in blood pressure when they take in moderate or large amounts of sodium, the component in table salt that we measure and monitor. As we said earlier, even if a person is not particularly salt sensitive, blood pressure still falls when sodium intake falls. But is it all about salt?

There are other elements in the diet, often called nutrients, that can affect blood pressure. Some interesting studies in the 1990s showed that many people are missing certain nutrients in their diets. It turns out it's not only about what you eat, but also what you *don't* eat (Thorogood, Hillsdon, and Summerbell 2003).

It turns out that calcium, magnesium, and potassium are important elements that often get left out of today's diets or are consumed in only small amounts. A diet that is high in refined or processed foods is low in these nutrients. You might remember from chapter 2 that sodium content is high in packaged foods such as crackers, chips, and pretzels. Sodium is also high in ketchup and most canned soups. Pickles are particularly high in sodium because they are "pickled" in brine, another name for salt water. By purposely moving away from these foods and eating more fruits and vegetables, you reduce sodium intake and increase magnesium, potassium, and calcium. Low-fat dairy items are a particularly good source of calcium.

Saturated Fat

Fats come in three main categories. *Saturated* fat is found in butter, lard, cream cheese, and coconut oil (also called palm oil on the containers of many foods). These are fats that raise your cholesterol and clog your arteries.

Polyunsaturated and *monounsaturated* fats are the other types of fats. More of the fats you eat should come from the monounsaturated (olive oil, canola oil) and polyunsaturated (corn oil, safflower oil) categories. A recent controversy has popped up because health experts have been recommending monounsaturated fats over polyunsaturates. It appears that some of the studies these recommendations are based on may have had design flaws, so throwing out safflower oil in favor of olive oil may not be right. Do reduce saturated fat, though. It's highly recommended that you limit your total daily calories from saturated fat to less than 10 percent, and less than 30 percent from fats in general. Fats have more calories, ounce for ounce, than other foods. If you eat more calories and don't burn them off, you'll gain weight. When your body weight goes up, your blood pressure goes up.

The DASH Diet

The DASH (Appel et al. 1997) study was a U.S. government–sponsored research project conducted at four large medical centers (DASH stands for *D*ietary *A*pproaches to *S*top *H*ypertension). The scientists found that blood pressure was reduced with an eating plan that is low in saturated fat, cholesterol, and total fat, and high in fruits, vegetables, and low-fat dairy products. This eating plan also emphasized poultry, fish, nuts, and whole-grain products. This diet is low in red meat, sweets, and beverages containing sugar. As you might imagine, the DASH diet is rich in potassium, magnesium, and calcium, as well as protein and fiber.

Unlike many previous studies that were done predominantly on white males, the DASH study included many women and African-Americans. The researchers compared three eating plans, each of which had a fixed amount of sodium (3,000 mg). The first diet was a usual diet for many Americans. The second was similar, but had increased fruits and vegetables, and the third was the DASH plan, with specific servings of all of the groups and a limit of 2,000 calories per day.

The results of this study were really remarkable. The diets with extra fruits and vegetables and the DASH eating plan both dropped blood pressure significantly, especially in the participants who had higher blood pressure. Not only that, but these reductions were seen within two weeks. Everybody was sort of surprised to see how effective these diets were, so they did a second study where participants either consumed a typical American diet or the DASH diet, but this time both groups had a salt restriction. Once people were assigned to the American diet or the DASH diet, they were followed for a month with either a "normal" sodium intake, a moderate reduction of sodium (2,400 mg/day), or a significant salt reduction (1,500 mg/day).

This second study showed that reducing salt intake reduced blood pressure in *both* diet groups. The DASH group always had lower blood pressure than the other group. The biggest blood pressure drop was seen in the DASH group consuming only 1,500 milligrams of sodium per day. Again, those with high blood pressure showed the biggest drop, but those with normal blood pressures also had a large decrease. So whatever your diet is now, your blood pressure will likely drop if you cut your sodium intake. And if your blood pressure is up, you'll get a lot more "bang for your buck" if you limit your salt and follow the DASH diet.

For more information on lowering your blood pressure with the DASH diet, visit the National Heart, Lung, and Blood Institute's Web site, http://www.nhlbi.nih.gov/health/public/heart/hbp/dash/introduction.html, or call (301) 592-8573 and ask for publication #06-4082.

Here are a couple of other tidbits before we leave this discussion on diet. A study from the Brigham and Women's Hospital in Boston (Winkelmayer et al. 2005) showed that blood pressure went up in women who drank more than four cola beverages per day (diet or regular), but no hypertension developed in women who got their caffeine from drinking coffee instead of cola. Because doctors have known for a long time that coffee consumption raises blood pressure in the short run (right after drinking it), they also assumed that it contributed to the development of hypertension. This interesting study casts some doubt on that, and raises concerns about excessive cola-beverage consumption.

And you're going to love this—having a small amount of dark chocolate (one ounce) might help, since the dark version has twice the amount of flavonoids found in milk chocolate. *Flavonoids* are chemicals found in the skins of dark fruits, red wine, and dark beer that can help to dilate blood vessels. But keep your chocolate consumption to a small amount to avoid excess fat and sugar. Both of these areas (caffeine and chocolate) should be fertile for more research. You may wish to volunteer.

All of these dietary details are important, but they become "trees" in the bigger "forest" of lifestyle changes that can help you maintain lower blood pressure. You don't want to lose sight of the forest for the trees.

Exercise

Regular exercise is good for you in so many ways. It feels good. It helps to reduce your weight (even a ten-pound weight loss can lower blood pressure). It changes your metabolism. It also blunts big swings in blood pressure seen in inactive or deconditioned people, often known as "couch potatoes." It even improves your mood.

The important thing about exercise is that it should be done *regularly*. That means almost every day. Everyone has days when they just can't make time for it, but if your rule of thumb is to exercise every day, then it isn't so bad if you miss a day or two here and there. And you should exercise for

thirty minutes or more a day. Simple walking is just fine —
you don't have to try out for the Olympics! Often doctors will
advise their patients to walk fast enough that it is just slightly
difficult to speak in a normal conversational voice. Swim-
ming and biking are also great because they avoid wear and
tear on the joints. All of these are good examples of *aerobic*
exercise, the most important kind for cardiovascular fitness
and lowering blood pressure.

The other type of exercise is called *isometric* exercise.
Heavy weight lifting is a good example of this type of exercise, and is generally not recommended if you have hypertension. If you have to grunt while you do it, it's probably
isometric. Lighter weights with more repetitions should be
fine, though, and can also help with flexibility.

Both diet and exercise can be challenging issues, even
for me, Dr. Bruce Wilson, one of the authors of this book. I'm
chronically struggling with building enough regular exercise
into my day or my week. My job as a physician doesn't
require me to move around very much. I love to play tennis,
and do so regularly, but a couple of years ago I developed a
painful foot condition called plantar fasciitis. Lots of people
get this, and regardless of all the medicines, injections, and
physical therapy you get, it just takes a long time to go away.
I was off my tennis schedule for more than a year, and had a
hard time doing any exercise. When it finally went away, I
got back to the court and promptly hurt my elbow — undoubtedly from being deconditioned. Eventually I had to stop playing again to let my elbow heal. By not cutting back on my
diet when I was unable to play tennis, I gained about twelve
pounds and felt like the Goodyear blimp.

Now that I'm back playing tennis again, I feel better, but
I have a hard time committing time every day, or most days,
to regular, aerobic exercise. I can almost always find an

excuse, especially when I'm traveling, which is frequently. So I'm just like most everyone. But I remind myself all the time that both diet and exercise are important. Stewing over them or feeling stressed or guilty about not living up to my diet or exercise plans just makes things worse. Staying emotionally balanced is probably the most important lifestyle change that you can make. As you'll see in the next chapter, emotional stress is a big contributor to high blood pressure. The HeartMath techniques in the last section of this book will help you develop the emotional balance you need to gain more control over lifestyle issues and the changes you want to make.

Smoking

The nicotine in cigarette (and also cigar and pipe) smoke causes a faster heartbeat and constricts blood vessels, both of which cause blood pressure to go up, at least temporarily. Smoking also causes the platelets in your blood, whose job it is to stick to the walls of blood vessels to start the process of blood clotting if you get a cut, to stick to cholesterol plaques on the insides of the coronary arteries that feed the heart. The platelets then become involved in the process of making the plaques grow. On occasion, the platelets can trigger a blood clot in an artery, which could block it off completely and cause a heart attack. Everybody knows that cigarettes cause cancer as well as emphysema and many other health problems. If you are a smoker and need help quitting, call the Quitline of the American Cancer Society at (800) ACS-2345.

Stress

In most books and articles about hypertension, there is usually only a paragraph or two about stress. That's mostly due to the fact that stress had not been measurable in the past. Yet most people feel that stress is contributing to their high blood pressure, and then the stress of the struggle to manage it also weighs on them. Dr. Stewart Wolf was one of the first researchers to examine the role of stress in hypertension, in his seminal book *Life Stress and Essential Hypertension* (1955, Williams and Wilkins).

We have a lot of compassion for the stress most people feel today. Tremendous progress has been made over the last ten or fifteen years to understand the underpinnings of stress. That's why Doc Childre, one of the authors of this book, started the nonprofit Institute of HeartMath, to research the mechanisms of mental and emotional stress and find solutions. The science behind stress has led to the development of effective tools to help people change their stress habits. Let's take a journey together and learn what your stress "wiring" is doing to you, and what you can do to reprogram it.

Chapter 6

Stress and Hypertension

Well, now we're down to the core issue, aren't we? Thus far we have defined normal blood pressure and hypertension. We've looked at other diseases that cause high blood pressure, as well as things that contribute to it. We spent some time going over medications and lifestyle changes that can help to bring blood pressure down. It's time now to tackle the mysteries of *stress.*

Our View of Stress

The definition of stress seems like it might be a little different from person to person. After all, stress for one individual might be a fun and exciting challenge for another. Some people are a complete wreck when they have to give a speech in front of a crowd, while others relish the chance to get on the stage and perform.

What are you actually *feeling* when you experience stress? Emotions are central to this experience for everyone; typically feelings such as tension, worry, anxiety, irritation, frustration, anger, lack of control, or helplessness have been triggered when people say they "feel stressed." Research done at the Institute of HeartMath has clearly shown that

> while thoughts and mental processes clearly play a role in stress, it is unmanaged disturbed emotions that provide fuel for its sustenance. It is also emotions — more than thoughts alone — that activate the physiological changes composing the "stress response." ... A purely mental activity, such as mentally recalling a past situation that provoked anger, does not produce nearly as profound an impact on psychological processes as actually engaging the emotion associated with that memory — actually re-experiencing the feeling of anger. (Rein, Atkinson, and McCraty 1995)

So it appears that the psychological effects of negative emotions contribute heavily to the effects of stress on the brain and body (McCraty 2006).

Most people spend a lot of time worrying or complaining about specific events that have occurred in the past, are bothering them in the present, or might be coming up in the future. Troubling news, problematic weather, difficulties with personal finances, the overgrown lawn, or a poor grade on your daughter's history exam are all events that may be labeled as "stress-causing." Add to that the traffic jam, the lady in front of you in the grocery store checkout line who is writing a check but forgot her driver's license, and your adolescent son who has found that challenging your ideas, appearance, or anything else is a sport. You may believe that if something could just be done about these problems, then life would get better and you'd have less stress. Oftentimes, however, thoughts and feelings associated with stressful events play over and over in your mind until they become *habitual*. Eventually, you can't even identify a specific event that triggered the ongoing anxiety or anger.

That Was Then, This Is Now

Daily living used to have fewer events and was a lot less complicated. Now, so much is going on at the same time, pressing in on people from all sides. Some refer to current times as the "information age." Everyone is bombarded with more and more information and complexity.

Recall how stressed many of us felt even back in the 1980s, before cell phones and e-mail. Now the information flowing through the galaxy is incessant. People can reach you anywhere, anytime, so they do. Your e-mail in-box fills up just as soon as you finish with the last batch. And have you noticed that the mere appearance of certain names in your in-box or your voice mail is enough to trigger your emotions? Most people we know feel like they've got information over-load and there's no shutting off the faucet—there's no down-time. And they feel there's not much they can do about it. It's the feeling of overload and lack of control—over issues and events—that creates and accumulates stress.

Looking more deeply at the problem, we'd like to introduce a more scientific definition of stress.

Stress is the emotional and physiological reaction to a perceived threat, whether real or imagined, resulting in a series of adaptations by the body.

From this scientific view, stress really isn't all the stuff that happens to you day in and day out. Stress is your reaction to it.

The Human Stress Response

Let's examine, for a moment, how the stress response developed over time. It's believed that humankind first showed up on this planet somewhere around 100,000 to 200,000 years ago. It was a different place back then. There were lots of physical threats to people as they walked through the jungle. Some paleontologists might argue about whether humans inhabited the Earth at the same time as the saber-toothed tigers, but that species makes a good example of a very real threat.

Imagine walking through the jungle and happening across a saber-toothed tiger and two of her cubs. That tiger sees you as a wonderful lunch for the family. It would be extremely beneficial for you to have an automatic reaction system built into you so that you might, if you were really lucky, run like the blazes and escape. To put it another way, your statistical chances of survival would be much greater if you had an automatic switch that would immediately activate your system in a number of ways to help you to avoid becoming the tiger's lunch.

Luckily, humans have just such a system. The *autonomic nervous system* (ANS) is the part of your nervous system that's automatic—"autonomic" is just another name for automatic. This part of the nervous system requires no thoughts or calculations—it kicks in immediately when you are faced with a threat to your survival. The autonomic nervous system has two branches.

The Sympathetic Nervous System

The *sympathetic* branch of the autonomic nervous system is frequently called your "fight-or-flight" system. This term was coined by Dr. Walter Cannon, a physiologist working in the beginning of the last century who was widely considered the godfather of stress research. We now commonly use this phrase to describe what happens when the sympathetic nervous system is activated. When faced with a physical threat, this system is turned on in a fraction of a second to prepare you to either fight the enemy or flee from it. Depending on what or whom you encounter, and under what circumstances, one of these two responses would be most appropriate. If a person half your size kicks you in the shin, you may stay and fight. But if you're looking eye-to-eye with a tiger, it's more advisable to take your chances with a rapid escape.

With either response, an entire cascade of events occurs faster than you could say "Holy %$@#!" The nerves in the brain quickly send signals along the nerves in your body that constrict your blood vessels, immediately raising your blood pressure. Your heart rate jumps up so your body can pump more blood to your muscles and you can run faster. Arteries in your skin constrict, making it less likely that you'll bleed to death if the tiger bites you. Blood is directed away from organs that really aren't necessary while you're running for your life, such as your kidneys and your digestive tract. You certainly don't want to be wasting your energy digesting the breakfast you ate this morning when your muscles need to use that oxygen-rich blood to get you out of there! Your pupils dilate so you might see a few more things (like that tree branch just ahead) while you're running. The hair on the back of your neck stands up so you might feel more elements in your surrounding environment. Again, it takes only parts of a second for all these elements of the sympathetic nervous system to spring into action.

The Parasympathetic Nervous System

The *parasympathetic* branch is the other arm of the ANS. Its function dominates when there's nothing perceived as threatening in your environment. Imagine yourself relaxed on the couch, watching a rerun of an old movie and eating popcorn. You have very little sympathetic activity playing in your nervous system now, and the parasympathetic arm is running the show. Blood is preferentially being delivered to your stomach and intestines to help you absorb and digest your food. Your heart rate is probably a little slower than usual, because you have no need for it to be fast. Your blood pressure is also lower. You're relaxed.

But suddenly there's a loud ring from the telephone right next to you. You jump about three inches, your heart starts pounding, and you feel sweaty. See how fast that was? You grab for the phone and calm yourself, realizing it's not a tiger (or a burglar alarm) but just a friend calling to chat. Soon that sympathetic jolt is withdrawn as you realize there's no physical threat, and the parasympathetic arm returns things to normal.

Remember our definition of stress: the emotional and physiological reaction to a perceived threat, whether real or imagined, resulting in a series of adaptations by the body. That phone ringing a moment ago wasn't a threat at all, but it startled you when you weren't expecting it. Have you ever been walking down a dark street at night and noticed a shadow that, at first, seemed like a mugger? In those first few moments before you realize it is just a shadow, the perceived or imagined threat acts just as powerfully to activate your fight-or-flight response as a real mugger would have. If you spent time in rational thought about whether that was a mugger or just a shadow, you might be without your wallet before you realized it. So it's good that your alarm system is activated immediately.

To understand stress, it's important to recognize how fast these swings in the autonomic nervous system take place.

Have you ever been driving your car along a quiet residential street when a young child rides his bike down a driveway and out in front of your car? Did you notice how fast that prickly sensation spread all over your skin, and how quickly your heart was pounding? These alterations in sympathetic and parasympathetic functioning occur very rapidly because whether it's a tiger, a mugger, or a kid on a bike, your ability to react is directly related to how fast your "switch" is thrown.

A Slower Set of Changes — The Hormonal System

In recent years, scientists have learned about a second stress-response system. This is a cascade of events referred to as the *neurohormonal* response because it's a long series of reactions involving nervous-system signals to many glands all over the body. These signals cause the production and release of hormones to increase your chance of survival during times of threat. These changes take a few minutes to get started, and may last minutes to hours.

Imagine now (you won't like this) that the saber-toothed tiger catches you. In most instances your survival mechanisms no longer matter, because you are now lunch. But just suppose that your fellow tribesmen spear the tiger after just one little bite on your leg. Once you're wounded, but not dead, you need a system to help you survive. Your hormonal system is going to provide you with some neat tricks. Its cascade of chemical steps is about 1,400 reactions long. These complex reactions can do many things. We'll take a look at a couple of the major ones.

Cortisol

Cortisol is known by some as "the mother of all stress hormones." That's because cortisol is released in large quantities when you perceive or feel stress. We talked in chapter 2 about the adrenal glands on top of the kidneys, how they produce adrenaline (also known as epinephrine), and how adrenaline can raise blood pressure. While adrenaline is produced in the central core of the adrenal gland, cortisol is produced in one of the three outer layers. Once it is released into the bloodstream, one of cortisol's main actions is to raise blood sugar or glucose. It does so by helping to break down stored sugars from places like your liver and your muscles. It's critical that your blood sugar stays high enough because the brain only knows how to use one type of "fuel," and that's glucose. The rest of your body also needs glucose to be readily available as an energy source.

Back to our story. A tiger just bit you, remember? Since it's unlikely that you'll be able to get to a mango tree for a sugar rush any time soon, your body will need to break down its stored sugars to make glucose so your brain can think about what to do next. Your muscles will need more fuel to respond. So, it's a neat design of nature to have a built-in cortisol system to raise blood sugar.

What else does cortisol do? Both directly and indirectly (by interacting with other hormones) it raises blood pressure by causing constriction of the arteries and interacting with the kidneys to save salt and water. (Remember that these functions also elevate blood pressure.) That seems like a rather bright idea right about now because you-know-who just bit your leg, and if you're bleeding away on the river bank, your blood pressure is dropping. When blood pressure gets dangerously low and can't push the right amount of blood to your organs, you'll go into shock. When shock comes from hemorrhage, or heavy bleeding, it's called *hemorrhagic* shock. So cortisol does a couple of key things to help you survive—it raises blood sugar and raises blood pressure. These responses to the "stress" of a tiger biting you sound like a great idea. Hold that thought.

Cortisol and Emotions

There are a couple of other important things you should know about cortisol. This potent hormone is also triggered by any negative emotion, such as anxiety, anger, or hostility, as well as depression. There's a feedback loop at work, too. Just as a bad mood triggers stress and cortisol release from your adrenal glands, that same cortisol, if it hangs around in your bloodstream for a while, can help to create a bad mood. We refer to this as a vicious cycle, because it feeds on itself. Bad mood triggers cortisol, which then makes you feel bad emotionally, which ends up creating more cortisol, which then makes you feel worse. If this feedback loop goes on long enough, you can feel submission and despair. Some call it "burnout." This is one of the reasons that chronic stress from events that you repeatedly respond to with emotions like worry, anxiety, or anger can lead to depression. It's not bad to have these emotions trigger cortisol—it is a necessary part of survival physiology. It's the inability to let go of them that keeps cortisol pumping through your system, causing burnout and depression. Chronic stress also leads to lack of mental clarity. Dr. Robert Sapolsky, a stress researcher at Stanford University, discusses this at length in his book *Why Zebras Don't Get Ulcers* (1998). Other scientists have also reported on the effects of cortisol on a multitude of sites in the brain, including inhibition of the ability to remember or think clearly (Newcomer et al. 1994).

DHEA

Before you experience despair just from reading this, take heart! (Ooh — great line — we're getting close to the best part.) Nature has a habit of keeping everything in balance. There's a yin and a yang in almost every system. That little adrenal gland has a whole bunch of other tricks up its sleeve, but probably the coolest one is the production of another hormone called DHEA. Since those letters don't make a word, they must stand for something long and complicated: *dehydroepiandrosterone* (no pronunciation help needed, since not even the scientists who work on this stuff every day call it anything other than DHEA).

DHEA is more difficult to explain because it hasn't been studied for as long or in as much depth as cortisol, its adrenal cousin. DHEA seems to counteract some of the effects of cortisol. Although cortisol is a necessary hormone for every-day function, by providing DHEA to counteract cortisol, it's as if Mother Nature knew that you were only supposed to get an extra dose of cortisol every now and again, and only in times of real danger when there's a physical threat to your survival. It's good to limit your exposure to things like tigers.

DHEA and Emotions

Just as cortisol production can be triggered by negative emotions, DHEA production can be related to positive emotions, such as happiness, love, care, gratitude, and appreciation. Conversely, DHEA can help create those same uplifting feelings while it's running through your bloodstream. As opposed to the vicious cycle described earlier for cortisol, DHEA seems to be at the center of a "virtuous cycle," because DHEA helps create positive mood, and positive mood helps create more DHEA.

DHEA has created a fair amount of controversy in the last ten years. While it's fair to say that it has beneficial effects when released naturally, there is more than a little concern about taking it as a supplement or as a treatment. While cortisol is an end product (it doesn't go on to become something else later), DHEA can be converted to one of the sex hormones, estrogen or testosterone. So taking a DHEA supplement can create side effects related to the sex hormones, such as facial hair in women or prostate enlargement or stimulation of prostate cancer in men.

There has been interest in DHEA as a vitality booster or an antiaging compound, which comes from the knowledge that DHEA is associated with positive mood. DHEA is produced in only very small amounts up until the age of six or seven years, then it's turned on and produced in large quantities up until the thirties or so. As you age, DHEA gradually declines so that by around age seventy-five it's only at about 25 percent of the level it was fifty years earlier. It's obvious that young children and people over seventy-five feel positive emotions, even though their bodies don't make much DHEA, so it's not a necessary component of these feelings. There are many other factors that contribute to positive and uplifting emotions, most of which have to do with the heart, which we will address later on. Nevertheless, people have wondered if taking DHEA supplements later in life could provide a "fountain of youth" of good feeling and better health. Athletes take it as a "performance hormone" in hopes of doing better in competition, but, as with any steroid, if it's discovered in their system the athletes will be disqualified.

There haven't been many long-term studies on the effects of taking DHEA supplements. While mice have been studied a little more, mice aren't humans. And the number of people studied has been quite small. Researchers who studied DHEA with high hopes for the DHEA pill are now the very ones warning people against taking it because of the side effects they have seen. Many are quite worried that DHEA shouldn't be a supplement at all because of its potent hormone effects, but be available only as a prescription drug for those with DHEA deficiency. It's not that there isn't excitement about this hormone, but until more is known about it, we recommend that your body be in charge of producing your DHEA and rebalancing your system. And there are ways to naturally increase your body's production of DHEA.

The World in the Twenty-First Century

All of this time spent on what adrenal glands do—why they greatly increase cortisol when your survival is threatened and why they make more DHEA when times are good—is leading to the core issue. While it's essential that your body crank up adrenaline and cortisol if a tiger is nibbling at your heels, the truth of the matter is that for most people, there aren't many tigers today.

Not that there are *never* any tigers—after all, you could fall over the railing at the zoo—but for the most part, modern culture is almost devoid of the ever-present physical threats of the past. There certainly are times when your life can be endangered, like a drunk driver crossing the median and bearing down on you at 60 miles per hour. Or you might be at an ATM machine when a guy with a gun approaches and demands your money. Or a natural disaster may be destroying your home and you need to get out fast. In those instances, it's essential to raise blood pressure. It's critical that you have a built-in system to squirt you full of adrenaline so you react very quickly. If that car accident actually happened and you were severely injured, without cortisol you would die.

Aside from instances like the ones above, for most people in modern culture physical threats are few and far between. Yet the "stress button" is being pushed all the time by all sorts of things, and eventually it gets stuck in the "on" position.

When the Stress Button Gets Stuck

When was the last time you actually enjoyed a traffic jam? How did you feel last time you got the runaround by one of those phone answering systems that endlessly tells you to press different numbers depending on what you're calling about, then doesn't give a clear option for what you need? How do you feel after arguments with spouses or adolescent children, financial challenges, constant deadlines, information overload, home/work conflicts, difficult bosses, problematic employees—the list of "stress triggers" goes on and on. The sad fact is that all of these negative feelings trip your stress alarm system just as if you'd been cornered by a tiger. Most people are bathing in adrenaline and cortisol when they were only meant to get an extra squirt every now and then.

What are the consequences of this? There are many. Since this book is about hypertension, we'll focus on that. Stressful emotions activate the sympathetic nervous system, and then increase adrenaline to make your heart beat faster and your blood vessels constrict. Stressful emotions also trigger cortisol, which causes blood vessel constriction and salt and water retention in the kidneys. The result is elevation in blood pressure. It's not hard at all to see why chronic stress, resulting from an ongoing accumulation of all the little stress reactions, is a direct link to high blood pressure. No wonder it's called hyper-tension.

There are lots of other things that go wrong when you take a long hot bath in cortisol and adrenaline. Don't forget that the leading cause of death is heart disease. As we mentioned, cortisol also raises blood sugar. High blood sugar contributes to obesity, as well as abnormal cholesterol levels, which both contribute to coronary artery disease. If your blood sugar gets too high, or stays elevated, you develop diabetes. All these stress-induced factors combine to create the chronic diseases that are killing most people.

How odd, then, that the chemical reactions that naturally take place in the body, in an attempt to improve people's chances of living if they are threatened, are actually killing them. People are dying of their own survival mechanisms because the environment has changed drastically and stress is everywhere. How about that—dying of the body's own survival mechanisms. So what do you do?

Chapter 7

Resetting Your Thermostat

A thermostat typically has something to do with temperature, but here we are referring to resetting the controls for blood pressure.

There are little clusters of nerves in the heart and along the arteries coming out of the heart that sense pressure. These sensors relay information into the area of your brain that regulates a lot of basic functions: breathing rate, heart rate, and blood pressure. This part of the brain is quick to make changes because it is partly responsible for your survival.

These changes fall into the category of "reflexes." They occur almost instantaneously and without any input from the thinking part of your brain. The reflex that involves sensing pressure and then responding with instructions to change your heart rate and relax or constrict the blood vessels is referred to as your *baroreceptor reflex*. *Baro* is the latin root for "pressure," as in *barometer*, an instrument that measures atmospheric pressure.

Ever since the 1930s or so, researchers have found a number of factors that can reset blood pressure reflexes. When some people experience stress frequently, or for prolonged periods of time, their systems get used to the higher blood pressure that often comes with it. After awhile, the control systems and sensors recalibrate to this higher pressure. Once that happens, the system will do everything it can to maintain this higher level of blood pressure—its job is to regulate blood pressure around a set point that it thinks is normal. This mechanism of "resetting" is a common reason why scientists believe people develop hypertension. If your blood pressure is up often enough, or long enough, the new level seems normal and the reflex is reset in the brain.

The good news is that it doesn't take that long to recalibrate the system back down to a healthier normal. That's what HeartMath is all about—physically throwing that switch that will help reset the controls back to normal. Before we teach you how to do exactly that, we have a few stories about people just like you who have achieved great success with the HeartMath program.

Stories of Resetting Pressure Levels

My first experience with this happened right in the hospital where I (Dr. Bruce Wilson) practice cardiology. A young nurse of about twenty-three came to me one day and told me that her blood pressure had been elevated recently. She had recently been married, had a wonderful relationship with her new husband as well as her own family, and had begun to consider having a family. She loved her job and was not a high-stress type of person. I had seen her in many situations, and never saw her lose her cool or appear frustrated or unhappy.

I told her that I would prefer to teach her the HeartMath techniques than put her on medications, especially since she was considering pregnancy. But her pressure was quite high, and after doing some basic testing, I put her on a small dose of medication, which brought her pressure down nicely. I then worked with her on HeartMath.

Within two or three weeks her pressure normalized, and I was able to taper her off the medication entirely. She was impressed, as was her doctor (me!). Not all of my patients would be this easy, or drop in such a short period of time, but I was very encouraged; one for one in the success column.

Another doctor wrote to us saying that he'd been using the HeartMath tools to teach his patients how to lower their blood pressure:

> *One of my patients had uncontrolled hypertension (220/110), even with medication. She also had chronic insomnia. At her second session learning HeartMath, her blood pressure at the beginning of the session was 200/110; at the end of session it had dropped to 130/70. I sent her home with HeartMath tools to practice. I also told her to purchase a home blood pressure monitor to record her readings twice a day while practicing HeartMath. When I saw her for her two-week follow-up, her daily blood pressure readings were all 130/70 to 140/80. She was also sleeping through the night for the first time in years, despite having taken prescription sleeping medications all those years.*

It's known that negative emotional states can produce stress, which can then lead to higher blood pressure. One study found that "people who say they are feeling anxious or depressed are two to three times more likely to go on to develop high blood pressure than calmer, happier individuals" (Jonas, Franks, and Ingram 1997, 45). Drs. Louise Hawkley and John Cacioppo at the University of Chicago have been studying loneliness for a long time. They published a study in 2006 that found that loneliness in people nearing retirement age was associated with higher blood pressure. Chronic feelings of social isolation were related to as much as a thirty-point rise in systolic blood pressure by the age of sixty-five, and this was independent of other risk factors (Hawkley et al. 2006).

> *R. W., a psychoanalyst, was very familiar with loneliness and social isolation in his patients. He had his own health problems as well. He was attempting to manage his own diabetes, hypertension, and obesity. He had tried numerous ways to manage all three, including prescription medications. R. W. succumbed to the same feelings of anxiety, guilt, and despair that he found in his own patients. He knew he needed something else to help him change the pattern. A doctor taught R. W. the HeartMath tools. After three months of practice, his diabetes came under control; he lost twenty pounds and his blood sugar fell from 300 to just over 100. His triglycerides dropped from over 500 to 100, and his blood pressure went from 150/78 to 130/84. More importantly, the HeartMath program allowed him to see he could control these conditions.*

In chapter 5, we talked about the recommended lifestyle changes to lower blood pressure. Most people with high blood pressure have heard all about these recommendations. We also talked about how hard it is for many people to succeed in making these changes. They may try some or all of them, but often can't seem to stick to a program. They often engage in "yo-yo" dieting and exercising, and feel tremendous anxiety and guilt when they don't follow through. Many people give up trying to fight against their bodies' set patterns. They feel helplessness and despair.

When Stress Becomes an Addiction

Stress in itself can become an addiction, just like food, alcohol, drugs, or gambling. Your baseline level for stress or any other addiction gets set into your system over time. Many people feel that they wouldn't know who they were if they weren't bathed in stress hormones all day. Stress addictions can shape your sense of identity.

> *J. B. is a forty-nine-year-old attorney with a tumultuous personal life and a very stressful law practice. He has high blood pressure and a very strong family history of heart disease. He suffered a massive heart attack and survived against heavy odds. HeartMath was part of his cardiac rehabilitation.*
>
> *During his training he learned how negative emotions impacted his underlying health. "But you don't understand, doctor," J. B. protested, "I deal with anger very well — I really blow my lid and get it out of my system, and then I'm done with it." J. B. was quite surprised to learn what was actually happening on the inside when he had his daily rants. He thought that he was actually helping himself by exploding. He didn't realize that he was sending his blood pressure sky high. J. B. came to realize that he was addicted to those outbursts, and with a little more insight, he admitted that they made him feel important.*

J. H., a high-tech entrepreneur, provides another example of stress getting wired into the body's hard drive:

> *I am a "hypertensive." I belong to the group which statistically makes up around 30 percent of the population. HeartMath helped me achieve control of my own hypertension and my addiction to stress.*

I was always going, going, going; taking that next cup of coffee to keep the adrenaline pumping while trying to keep my uncontrolled emotions from getting me in trouble in relationships. Now that I have learned to regulate my emotions and increase the percentage of positive emotions like care and appreciation flowing through my body, I don't have to take hypertension drugs at all anymore. The drop below my previous blood pressure levels was significant and I now experience clinically normal blood pressure. Over the years, I experimented with diet and exercise to see what effects they had on my pressure. I knew what effects coffee and smoking had had on my blood pressure, and while I found that diet and exercise regimens made a slight difference, they did not break the stress addiction. The HeartMath tools did. The emotional freedom gained has had a significant impact on my whole sense of well-being and on my relationships.

The Power to Change

The Institute of HeartMath found that there is a very special mode that the heart and cardiovascular system can shift into that helps give people the power they need to reset unhealthy baseline patterns. We will talk more about this mode in upcoming chapters. The important point now is to know that the HeartMath tools you will learn in chapter 9 were scientifically designed to help you shift into this empowered mode. Regular practice of tools to increase heart coherence has been shown to reset the baroreflex system (Lehrer et al. 2003) and lower blood pressure (McCraty, Atkinson, and Tomasino 2003).

Chapter 8

The Big Connection

Now that we've taken a look into how the body and emotions respond to all sorts of stress triggers, whether real or imagined, and read some case histories of people who have learned to reset their blood pressure "thermostats," it's time to delve into the HeartMath story. It provides some very exciting information that offers real hope. HeartMath research has everything to do with your heart, and how your heart talks to your brain.

The HeartMath Story, as Told by Founder Doc Childre

In the early 1970s I began researching the physiology of stress and emotions. I found that when people were under mental or emotional stress, they often perceived relationships and issues quite differently from when they were experiencing positive feelings, or were at peace with themselves and their lives. When people experienced genuine feelings of gratitude, care, appreciation, or even love, their perspective often widened and they intuitively saw how to resolve problems that were troubling them.

Back then there were no universities studying the effects of positive emotions on health and performance, as there are today. Hundreds of self-help books and courses were available that tried to teach people how to be happier. I found a common thread in many of these philosophies and traditions: fulfillment was said to exist "in the heart." I wanted to know if this was true.

Have you ever noticed that at times you "feel" strong emotions—either positive or negative—in the center of your chest? Many writers and artists have portrayed this observation in one way or another over the ages. Philosophers, poets, musicians, playwrights, and lovers throughout history have written or spoken of feelings that seem to come from the heart. The Latin word for heart is *cor*. The French word for heart is *coeur*. The Spanish word for heart is *corazón*. People today speak of "core" values that come from the heart. They use phrases all the time like "heartfelt emotions," or "heartbroken," or "put your heart into it," or "the heart of the matter."

I felt intuitively that there was a real and physical connection between the heart and emotions. I knew that my heart felt full when I was loving or appreciating someone, and my heart felt constricted when I was angry or hurt. I decided to expand my research to understand why this was so. So I delved into the field of neurocardiology, studying how the heart and brain work together, to see if I could figure out something about the "math" of the heart.

In 1991, I formed the Institute of HeartMath, a nonprofit research organization in Boulder Creek, California, to study the physiology behind what had been poetic lore for thousands of years. I assembled a team of psychologists, physiologists, and other scientists to build an electrophysiology laboratory to research the connections between heart and brain in greater depth than what was in the current literature. We gathered together a prestigious board of scientific advisors to guide our research. World-renowned psychiatrists, cardiologists, brain researchers, mathematicians, and physicists, along with engineers and biofeedback experts, helped design our study protocols and critique the incoming data. Here's a look at what we found.

Understanding the Power of the Heart

Scientists have known for many years that electromagnetic waves are generated by many structures in the body. Brainwaves are a good example. The machine that measures brainwaves is called the *electroencephalograph*, or EEG. Your stomach and intestines generate electromagnetic waves as they contract and relax at regular intervals. This helps to optimize the absorption of nutrients and water so you have the "fuel" to run the machinery of your body.

The heart's electromagnetic waves were first measured in 1903 with the development of the *electrocardiograph*, usually referred to as the ECG or EKG. A fact that can seem very surprising is that the heart's electrical signal (ECG) is actually about fifty times stronger (in electrical amplitude) than the brain's signal (EEG). Although this had been observed for over a hundred years, nobody wondered about the significance of it—until recently.

The observation that the heart's waves are stronger than the brain's sort of goes against how scientists and the rest of us view the human system. Most scientists have been taught that the brain controls everything. It therefore makes little sense that the signals coming from the heart would be so much stronger than the signals coming from the master control center, or that it would matter.

But that's what research is about—looking at the obvious and challenging assumptions. Scientists now have discovered that they can measure your heartbeat by detecting the heart's electromagnetic waves eight feet away from your body! On the other hand, if they want to measure your brainwaves using this same type of equipment, they can only detect them a couple of inches away from your head.

Scientists know that electromagnetic waves carry information. Radio waves are a common example of how information is sent out via electromagnetic waves. The waves that your heart and brain generate carry information that is sent through your body and out into the space around you, just like a radio transmitter. Yet the heart's signals have much more power.

A New Research Tool—HRV

Our HeartMath research team, headed by Dr. Rollin McCraty, wanted to know what the heart waves and brain waves were doing and saying. We learned that the heart and brain talk to each other in a number of ways, one of which is through the autonomic nervous system. We came upon a process that gave us a window into this conversation. By analyzing the patterns of *heart rate variability*, or HRV, which is derived from the ECG, we could see changes in people's mental and emotional states.

Everybody's heart rate varies. Of course it has to. When you are asleep, your heart beats slowly—maybe only about 50 or 60 beats per minute. When you're running up a hill, it might be beating at 160, or even higher, to help bring more blood to your leg muscles. So your heart beats as fast or as slow as it needs to beat. While the source of your heartbeat — your own built-in pacemaker — is right in the heart itself, the messages that regulate the speed of the heartbeat come down along nerves from the brain to the heart. Your heartbeat is independent of the brain, but it's modulated by, or influenced by, the brain. Your brain needs to vary the heart rate in order to meet the perceived demands of the moment, whether running from danger or lying perfectly still in bed.

You may be interested to learn that HRV technology isn't new; it's what's inside the fetal monitor of obstetrics units in every hospital. When a woman is having a baby, the doctors and nurses watch the baby's heartbeat. But it's not just the rate of the baby's heart — it's the pattern of how the heart rate is changing, or *varying*, that holds the valuable information. It tells the doctor whether the baby is in distress or whether everything is just fine.

Analyzing the HRV Pattern

The pattern of change in heart rate is analyzed by cardiologists to predict survival after a heart attack and survival in general (Stein et al. 2005). By analyzing the HRV pattern of change in a different way, the research team at HeartMath found that people's emotional states are also reflected in their HRV patterns (McCraty et al. 1995).

What do the patterns shown in figure 1 mean? These patterns are from the same person, recorded while she was experiencing different emotions. Notice the heart rate scale on the left of each of the recordings. The average heart rate is the same in both recordings, averaging about seventy beats per minute. But the top pattern shows the heart rate going up

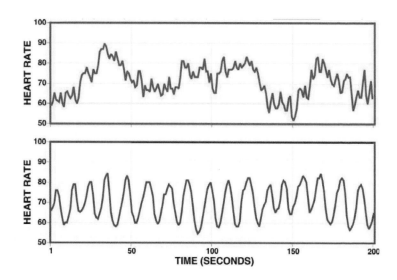

Figure 1: Patterns of heart rate variability (HRV)
The top panel demonstrates a very irregular pattern, known also as a chaotic pattern. The pattern on the bottom panel is very regular, or orderly, demonstrating a property known in physics as coherence.

and coming down in a very erratic pattern. "Herky-jerky" would be a very good way to describe it, wouldn't you say? Actually, when physics experts are analyzing wave forms like this, they use the term *chaotic* for the top pattern.

The bottom pattern has a very different look to it. When physicists see a very orderly pattern like the one seen on the lower graph, they use the term *coherence*. So the top pattern of changing heart rate is chaotic, while the bottom pattern is *coherent*.

Emotions and HRV

The significance of these two different patterns is striking as you watch them change in real time. We can attach a small, portable heart monitor to you and record your heartbeats and HRV patterns for twenty-four or forty-eight hours at a time. It's interesting to observe that a somewhat chaotic pattern is present almost all the time that you are awake and active. That's because your sympathetic and parasympathetic nervous systems are speeding up and slowing down the heart rate in order to meet the needs of the moment. However, when your stress response has been activated, or when you are experiencing negative emotions such as anger, hostility, or frustration, the pattern goes haywire and looks a lot like an earthquake graph. (Isn't that how you feel sometimes when you are emotionally upset?)

The coherent pattern can occur when you are in the most deeply relaxed stage of sleep. That makes sense, because your heart rate is gently fluctuating up and down, not being influenced by events or emotions, while your body is in the process of regenerating itself. But the coherent pattern occasionally is seen also during the time you are awake. Why?

The HeartMath research team made a rather astounding observation. We found that the coherent pattern is often seen when you are feeling sincere, positive emotions, even while you are active. It's also found during times of peak performance, even when your heart rate is very high. The coherent pattern isn't generated by low heart rate or relaxation, it is generated by how you feel (McCraty et al. 1995). People have used a number of terms for this coherent state—"being in sync," or "in a positive flow," or "in the zone." Everyone falls into the zone from time to time, usually inadvertently. Professional athletes seem to experience this more than most, but the zone also can occur when you are working, communicating, or creating. It's characterized by clarity, a sense of timelessness, effortlessness, and positive mood.

The Three Levels of the Human Brain

As animals evolved, they developed three layers in the brain. The first layer, present in virtually all animals, has survival functions in it. This first brain resides at the top of the spinal column, just inside the skull, at the back. The centers in this area of the brain regulate breathing, heart rate, blood pressure, and many other functions necessary for keeping the body alive. Obviously, these are all very automatic functions — you don't have to think about how fast your heart should be beating or how many times a minute to breathe. This part of the brain in humans is often called the "hindbrain" because it's in the back.

The second layer that developed is known as the "midbrain." Certain structures in this midbrain, which sits on top of the hindbrain, have complex connections that deal with emotion and memory. Together, these elements of the midbrain make up what is called the *limbic system*. One structure in the limbic system is particularly interesting because it acts as an emotional memory scanner. It's called the *amygdala* (uh-MIGG-dah-lah). The amygdala is always scanning what's going on in your experience right now, and comparing it to all the events in your emotional memory bank. Even if you have repressed a memory because it may have been unpleasant, the amygdala will react to what's happening to you at this moment based on what you have experienced before.

The reason the amygdala is so important is that it serves as the general alarm button for your entire system. Suppose you are walking down a street late at night by yourself. That might be a little frightening, depending on what city you're in. As you turn a corner, there's a large shadow just to your right.

Let's pause this movie for just a moment. If you have lived in very safe places your whole life, and still do, there might not be anything at all in your emotional memory bank that looks like this. But suppose you were once held up at night at gunpoint, or were frightened in another way in a similar situation. Your amygdala remembers that feeling and its association with that experience.

So now that you're in potentially similar circumstances, your amygdala is probably sending warning signals to your system. When you round that corner and see a shadow—full alert! The amygdala triggers your entire brain and nervous system to go into survival mode. As mentioned earlier, there are about 1,400 biochemical reactions that start to take place. The sympathetic nervous system immediately is activated for "fight or flight." Adrenaline spills into your system, further raising your heart rate and blood pressure. Shortly thereafter cortisol shows up, raising your blood sugar and your blood pressure to prepare you for the danger that you sense.

Pattern Matching

The notion of a left brain and right brain with entirely separate functions is fading. Researchers now realize that it's not quite as simple as one function coming from one side of your brain, and another coming from the opposite side. There's a lot of crossover. Dr. Karl Pribram, while head of the Neuropsychological Laboratory at Stanford University, found that the brain acts much more like a pattern recognition machine (Pribram and Melges 1969). It is always looking for a pattern to match to a previous experience or situation. Familiar situations that have been positive experiences do not set off your alarm system. But if that amygdala matches what's happening right now to something that has had a bad outcome in the past, ding! ding! ding!—your survival physiology is activated. You see, this emotion and memory pattern recognition in your limbic system has a lot of advantages to it. The faster you can match a pattern for danger, the more likely you will react to it and avoid harm—physical or psychological. Positive associations are also stored in this limbic system, so recognizing the earmarks of a pleasurable, caring, or nurturing situation is important, too, because you'll be drawn to it.

The Top Layer—The Cerebral Cortex

Let's get back to those three layers of the brain. People are different from all other animals in that humans developed a huge layer of gray matter on top of the other two. This layer is called the *cortex* (cover, or cap). While many other animals have a cerebral cortex, the human brain is about 80 percent cortex. Higher order brain functions occur up on top. Your ability to think, reason, calculate, learn, speak languages, do math, and many other complex functions resides up here in the executive suite. One of the big advantages of this part of the brain is that it allows you to ponder what might happen in the future. It's where foresight and planning come from. Perhaps most importantly, you form opinions and judgments because of this layer. All of this depends on that big cortex on top.

The Heart-Brain Connection

Now that we've reviewed what happens in each of the three layers of the brain, let's get back down to the heart. But before we do that, pause for a moment to recall key points from earlier in this chapter:

- The electromagnetic signal of the heart (ECG) has about fifty times more amplitude than your next biggest signal generator — the brain (EEG).

- Your heart signals can be measured about eight feet away from your body, while your brain signals can be measured only at or near your brain's surface.

- Heart rate variability (HRV) technology allows doctors and scientists to see how your heart and brain are communicating.

- Your heart rate patterns (HRV) reflect your emotional state. The chaotic pattern is seen during periods of stress and negative emotion. The coherent pattern is seen during periods of sincere, positive emotion and when you're "in the zone."

Now let's add to this summary a relatively new discovery in the field of neurocardiology: The information being sent north from heart to brain is far more abundant than the amount of information going south from brain to heart. (Cameron 2002). Once again, this violates the basic assumption that most people were taught: that the brain controls everything. Let's look a little deeper.

The signals ascending from the heart go up to the survival centers in the hindbrain where blood pressure, heart rate, and respiratory rate are controlled. This part of the brain analyzes the incoming information and makes changes

("Breathe faster, dummy — your oxygen is getting low!"). But there's more.

These very powerful heart signals affect not only these most basic functions. They also affect your feelings and your emotional memory center in the midbrain, the amygdala. In fact, the cells of the amygdala synchronize to the pacemaker cells in your heart (Frysinger and Harper 1990). So if your HRV pattern is highly chaotic, the amygdala often matches that to a negative emotional experience and automatically recalls that negative feeling. Your brain waves up in the cortex are also affected by those powerful chaotic heart signals, coloring how you think and perceive (Sandman, Walker, and Berka 1982). Your heart signals reach all the way to the top, altering all of those complex functions (van der Molen, Somsen, and Orlebeke 1985). So your executive-level processing, such as calculation, communication, planning, and creativity, is affected by the pattern the brain is recognizing from the big signal generator below — the heart.

That seemed totally upside down to scientists — but it's true, and it makes a lot of common sense to people who have learned to "listen to their hearts." The beauty of research is that it eventually reveals what had been overlooked or misunderstood in the past. Rather than being shocked by these new findings, it's time to see how to put them to work.

Chapter 9

The HeartMath Tools

You can learn to shift your emotions and change your HRV pattern to reverse stress and improve your health. Dr. Grant Slinger, director of Keystone Wellness Clinic in Rockefeller Plaza, New York, and a licensed HeartMath provider, teaches his patients how to do just that.

> *A. P. was referred to Keystone Wellness by his primary care physician because he was hypertensive, obese, prediabetic, and unable to lose weight. A highly successful owner of a company in the high-stress construction industry, A. P. had a lot of anxiety and anger. He harbored a kitchenette and vending machine in his private office, where he ate chocolate bars and other goodies. When he went to a restaurant, he couldn't resist emptying the entire bread basket. A. P. had tried controlled eating plans, but was unable to follow them. He knew what to do but couldn't stick to it. He knew that a lot of his problem was due to the stress he was under. He was in fear for his health, which he knew was in danger.*
>
> *"When A. P. came to us, his blood pressure was 160/80," Dr. Slinger reported. "We explained how the HeartMath program works and that he did have*

*control over changing his HRV. That was a big 'aha'
for him. He decided to use the HeartMath program
without messing around. After his first session, he felt
much better and his family commented that he seemed
more at ease. A. P. said that using the HeartMath
tools to change his HRV pattern to the coherent mode
interrupted his thought and emotion process. After five
training sessions at the clinic, he found that he was
becoming more aware of what he was eating and had
more control over it, even in the midst of difficult
business decisions. In just over three months, he lost
thirty-eight pounds and his blood pressure dropped to
120/70. This time period included the holiday season,
when the temptation to eat even more was greater.
His temperament changed completely. He was smiling,
and more relaxed overall. Recently, A. P. suffered the
loss of a family member. He was able to handle it
without returning to his old habits."*

Stress has been shown to be a very powerful component
of many diseases, not just hypertension. It may even be a
more powerful risk factor for heart disease than smoking,
blood cholesterol levels, or genetics. And in many cases,
reducing stress can help reduce these other risk factors.

*B. N. wrote: "My husband has seen a dramatic
decrease in his blood pressure (from 200s/100s to
90s/60s and 70s!) since he started using the
HeartMath tools two years ago. His cholesterol is
now less than 200 (it was close to 300). The tools
gave him insight into what coherence feels like, so
that when he feels his stress level rising, he can shift
into that state. His meds have been reduced and we
anticipate that he'll be able to discontinue them at*

*some point. We have also worked with his diet and
exercise, including yoga. This didn't seem to impact
the BP and cholesterol too much, perhaps because
there's a lot of genetics and family history with high
blood pressure and cholesterol. I can honestly say
that learning to shift out of stress in the moment
as it arises is what essentially changed his BP, his
cholesterol, and his life in a very positive way!"*

How Controlling HRV Can Reverse Stress

When an event occurs that triggers your stress response, nerve centers in your brain rapidly send signals to other areas of the brain to respond. At this point the response is unconscious, and you have not yet experienced the actual feeling. Signals are sent down the nerves to the heart, glands, and other organs and an entire cascade of 1,400 biochemical reactions is set into motion—all part of the alarm system. When these signals arrive at the heart, they create a chaotic HRV or heart rhythm pattern. Then this chaotic pattern is sent back up to the limbic centers in the midbrain that deal with emotion. The amygdala recognizes the chaotic pattern. This is when you actually "feel" the anxiety, panic, or anger.

Up in the executive suite of your cortex, these chaotic signals from the heart inhibit cortical function. The "smart" part of your brain shuts down to a degree. After all, you don't need to be able to do your calculus homework when you're being chased by a tiger. This turns out to be an explanation for why people do really stupid things when they're stressed out or badly frightened. Everybody certainly has had that experience.

Fortunately, the opposite is also true. When the HRV signal from the heart is coherent, the brain's three levels all synchronize and you experience what is called *cortical facilitation* (improved function). It's all systems go. Your field of perception is wider, your reaction times improve, and you see solutions more easily. You interpret events in the environment differently—more clearly; and you react in a more productive way—more intelligently. Now you know why Doc coined the term "heart intelligence."

Right about now you might be saying to yourself, "If these heart signals are so powerful, and the pattern they are sending up to the brain so profoundly influential over all these areas, wouldn't it be great to find a way to throw a switch so that coherence is being broadcast instead of chaos?

This is exactly what HeartMath is about. Now that you understand that chronic, recurrent stress signals are actually harming you in many ways, it would be far better for your blood pressure and your higher brain function if your big signal generator was singing the coherence song—unless your life is actually being threatened at the moment.

By using HRV technology, the researchers at the Institute of HeartMath were able to observe the changing rhythmic patterns of the heart while people experienced either stressful or positive emotional states. Once they saw that, all they had to do was experiment in their laboratory with different "triggers" that might help throw the coherence switch.

While many techniques developed over hundreds or even thousands of years (meditation, prayer, yoga, tai chi) can be effective, they often don't work immediately and can't be done in the moment. Don't forget that once that rapid stress response occurs, it can continue uninterrupted for long periods. As stated earlier, many people have become habituated to stress—it seems to be present most of the time. They need something to stop the stress reaction as soon as it starts— right now!

First Things First—Recognizing That Your Stress Button Has Been Pushed

If you are going to learn to stop your stress response and all of its consequences, you're going to have to be more in tune with how it feels when it has been activated. Many people experience this chemistry so much of the time that it has become white noise in the background. Some even say that it's normal to live like this—it's just the way the world is now.

It doesn't have to be this way. But if you're going to learn to throw your switch, you have to pay attention to your stressful feelings. Your internal radar screen has to become a little more sensitive, so you can know when your stress button has been pushed and then you can take steps to turn it off.

Neutral—The Most Basic Tool

The concept of *neutral* is not new. One of your mentors might have told you to "try to stay neutral." Neutral is a pretty good place to be. Think of the neutral gear in your car that allows you to pause and shift direction should the need arise. Neutral allows you to evaluate things more clearly and go in the best direction for the situation. It prevents you from reacting in a way that will bring you more trouble. If you're going sixty miles an hour, however, it's going to take you awhile to stop or slow down to neutral and change direction. Most people know exactly this feeling when they get into an argument or disagreement with someone they really care about. The emotions run high, and they blurt out something in the heat of the moment that they know they'll regret even as the words are passing through their lips. That little voice in the head says, "Oh no, I didn't just say that ... I wonder how long it's going to take to recover from that one?" In many situations people wish they could get to neutral faster. They can—by engaging the power of the heart first.

The Neutral Tool

Think of Neutral as a "time-out zone" where you can step back, neutralize your emotions, and see more options with clarity. The HeartMath Neutral tool has only two simple steps: Heart Focus and Heart Breathing.

Heart Focus

When you feel your stress button being pushed, recognize it. Then shift your attention from all that internal noise and chatter in your head down to the center of your chest—the area around your heart. (After all, if you're going to use this master pendulum, you'll need to engage it by focusing in that area.)

1. Simply let your attention drop gently down to your chest, and try to focus there. The next step will help you keep your focus in this area so you'll be able to maintain it.

Heart Breathing

Imagine that you are slowly breathing in and out through your heart. Of course, you can't actually breathe through your heart—that's what your lungs are for. But engaging your heart and using your imagination is very important to the process. So slow your breathing down a little. Count to five or six while you're breathing in through your heart—slowly and easily—and let it out to a count of five or six. This helps regulate your HRV. Now, gently, without extra work or effort, forget counting and just let the air come in and go out in that easy rhythm while you try to disengage from stressful thoughts and feelings.

2. Take a time-out; breathe slowly and deeply. Imagine the air entering and leaving through the heart area, or center of your chest. Try to disengage from your stressful thoughts and feelings as you continue to breathe. Repeat this a few times, keeping your focus right in the center of your chest until you've taken the charge out of the negative thoughts and emotions and you feel your stress response "neutralized."

Neutral is a great place to be. It stops the energy drain associated with all of that nervous-system traffic and complicated chemistry. It enhances brain function, giving you a range of choices that will help, not further complicate, your situation. Neutral is helpful even after the stress response has been triggered and you have reacted by doing something stupid that will bring you, and possibly others, more stress. At any point in the chain reaction, you can use the Neutral tool to stop it in its tracks. If you want your blood pressure to be lower, you will want to stop reacting in a way that keeps pumping all those stress chemicals into your system.

B. R. was diagnosed with malignant hypertension, the most severe form. B. R. says:

The doctors told me that I should have had a stroke and died. My blood pressure was 250/140 when I was admitted to the hospital. They couldn't do a stress test because my blood pressure was so high and they were going to give me an injection to do an invasive test. I remembered the HeartMath tools that I'd been taught but hadn't been practicing. I was lying on the gurney when I told them, "Give me fifteen minutes, I'll breathe through the heart and get it down." After fifteen minutes, I got it to 190/120 but it was still too high. After five more minutes of deeply focusing in my heart and heart breathing, it went down to 150/90 and my cardiologist was shocked. They put me on three medications and regular practice of HeartMath tools. I really learned to practice Neutral. I had to. Now, six months later, I have my blood pressure under good control.

Neutral is powerful. It changes the tune playing on your internal hard drive. In most situations, the Neutral tool takes less than a minute to be effective if you mean business. You can do it ten, twenty, even fifty times a day, just for practice. Then it can become an automatic response when you really need it.

But Neutral is only the first part of the process. The emotional charge is gone, but you may still be feeling anxiety or tension. You need to make an emotional shift. So let's take regulating your HRV one step deeper, so you can make this positive shift in the direction of not only less cortisol, but more DHEA.

Quick Coherence

Quick Coherence is a rapid three-step technique to shift your emotional state and have positive emotions running through your system. This helps you get the coherence pattern going on your big signal generator so that all of the functions in your body synchronize, and all the stress chemical pathways reverse. You've already learned the first two steps of Quick Coherence (Heart Focus and Heart Breathing); they're the same as the Neutral tool.

Now let's add the third step, Heart Feeling. In this step, you will engage a positive emotion to shift into coherence.

Back in the early 1990s, when the team of researchers at the Institute was experimenting with various triggers to switch over to coherence, they listened carefully to Doc's earlier research findings and personal experiences. He had found that intentionally generating sincere, positive feelings of love, care, gratitude, and appreciation gave people more mental clarity. These happen to be the same positive emotions that all the world's major religions have asked people to practice over hundreds and even thousands of years. Perhaps their founders intuitively knew that these positive emotions, sincerely felt, change the heart in some way.

That smooth, rhythmic, orderly pattern of coherence gets broadcast by your heart, your most powerful beacon. That signal goes north up to your brain, hitting the emotional centers in the midbrain, like your amygdala. This coherent pattern helps override negative emotional programming and gets transmitted all the way to the frontal lobes of your brain. That's when you can actually choose, with that smarter part of your brain, to respond more intelligently to the situation you're in. You experience cortical facilitation and are likely to see more appropriate ways to respond — ways that will bring you less stress, not more.

In the laboratory, the HeartMath scientists observed that the mood or emotion of appreciation seemed to be the easiest "switcher" of the HRV pattern over to coherence. While all genuine, positive emotions will do this, appreciation worked fastest for most people, most of the time. But again, any positive feeling will work if sincerely practiced. A positive feeling state is just that — a feeling. It's not a thought process. You want to genuinely feel the appreciation. If you can't feel appreciation (and some people can't at first), simply pick someone or something that you're grateful for, or care very much for, to appreciate. Even if you can't feel the feeling of appreciation, having the attitude of appreciation will start the process. This worked for M. H., a successful corporate lawyer with high blood pressure.

> *M. H. was overweight, pale, and couldn't look you in the eye. He was extremely unhappy and stressed and was classified as an emotional eater. He had been to doctors and knew everything he should be doing correctly, but he couldn't stick to it. He didn't think he could have control. After four months of practicing HeartMath and what he calls "appreciation attitude shifting," he stopped emotional eating and lost nearly 30 pounds, going from 296 pounds to 269 pounds. His blood pressure also went from 162/110 to 122/84, allowing his doctor to decrease his blood pressure medication by 50 percent. He is now much happier and more able to deal with stress. In his words, "It's spooky how differently I feel."*

When you're first learning the Quick Coherence technique, it can be helpful to remember a time or moment in your life that makes you feel good by just remembering it. See if you can pick one of those times right now. It doesn't matter what it is—a warm beach, a sunset, a mountaintop, being with someone you love, a pet, or even a favorite meal. It's not thinking about that experience that helps you get coherent, it's the actual feeling you have from recalling it. It's not a picture to be imagined—it's your positive emotional memory of the experience.

As you gain experience with the HeartMath tools, you will want to build a file of these positive moments in your past that you can recall when stress is triggered, to help you activate a positive feeling. Remember, you're switching feelings to get into coherence, not to get an A on a test. As you get into more coherence, you'll have more intelligence available to you on how to best respond to a situation.

What you'll find as you practice Neutral and Quick Coherence is that things that used to give you stress won't bring about those same reactions anymore. Those frenzied, reactive feelings will increasingly be replaced by more balance, calm, and clarity. That's because coherence is becoming a dominant pattern in your system more and more of the time. Your brain function is changing. You enjoy a broader field of perception, and you're more open to the many things going on all around you that bring you sincere appreciation. You develop a keen awareness of when you're coherent and when you're not. When your stress physiology is in gear, you'll notice that your field of vision is narrowed, as if you're looking through a straw, and only at "the enemy," not realizing that enemy is your own limited perception.

So it's time to try all three of the Neutral and Quick Coherence steps:

1. **Heart Focus** — Shift your attention to the area of the heart and breathe slowly and deeply.

2. **Heart Breathing** — Keep your focus in the heart by gently breathing — five seconds in and five seconds out — through your heart. Do this two or three times.

3. **Heart Feeling** — Activate and sustain a genuine feeling of appreciation or care for someone or something in your life. Focus on the good heart feeling as you continue to breathe through the area of your heart.

As you try to sustain this positive feeling, you'll find that your thoughts will wander or you'll be distracted by a phone ringing or voices nearby. That's okay. Simply return to the heart breathing, and after a few cycles in and out, reengage that positive feeling.

Neutral and Quick Coherence are the most basic tools, and the ones you'll need in order to switch out of the stress response that's raising your blood pressure, so that you can lower the pressure and keep it down. Frequent practice of these tools can take place almost any time or any place — while walking, driving, or even in the middle of a stressful conversation.

Coherence training isn't relaxation therapy. Relaxation is a state of low activity and can lead to drowsiness. Being able to relax is important, but you can be relaxed and still feel worried or depressed. Coherence, triggered by the orderly, rhythmic pattern in the signal from your heart, is associated with positive feelings and positive energy, as well as clear, efficient thinking that helps you interpret information with less bias. Creativity is enhanced and problem solving is simpler. That's why people sometimes call periods of sustained coherence "the zone." It's where they perform at their best. Coherence stops energy drain in the most physical sense. It builds the power to rewire your system to healthier and more efficient function.

Chapter 10

Rewriting Your Patterns

If we are going to help you rewire your system to change your blood pressure, we're going to have to help you rewrite your patterns and reset your thermostat. As stated earlier, many people get so bombarded by events and negative emotions that their system stays stuck in a negative pattern of responses. Those negative emotions create chaos, psychologically and physiologically, which can become so familiar that it feels normal. The greatest news is that by using your heart you can rewrite those patterns without as much time and effort as you may think.

Writing New Patterns

Do you remember learning how to drive? What an anxiety-provoking experience that was for most people! You had to learn each step. It required lots of cortical brain function. Your cognitive skills had to be used over and over: *Hold the steering wheel at ten o'clock and two o'clock. Put on your turn signal. Look over your left shoulder. Check the rearview mirror. Now check the side view mirror; now look over your shoulder again. Now change lanes. Prepare to turn left. Put on your turn signal again. Foot off the gas; now gently apply the brake. Now, hand-over-hand, turn the steering wheel. Now recover, back to straight again. Now more gas.*

Exhausting! And that was just learning how to make a turn. Ultimately you had to learn how to do something as complicated as parallel parking. It required lots of focus, and attention, and calculation, and experience, and repetition.

If you were asked today how you drive your car to work or to the grocery store, you'd probably name the route you take. But if asked specifically how you operate your car to get from point A to point B, you'd have no recollection of all those steps. Now you are able to drink your cup of coffee, answer your cell phone, and speak to the other person, all while driving a two-ton machine, often at high speeds and with multiple manipulations. And you get to work just fine. How does that happen?

After performing the same tasks over and over, repeating each step many times, these actions eventually become automatic. They are performed by a lower portion of your brain, saving your cognitive areas for matters such as evaluating driving conditions, or navigating through unfamiliar territory.

When actions become automatic, they have imprinted a pattern that has become familiar. Once this happens, messages are sent much more quickly and easily along the pathways of the nervous system. More traffic along the familiar pathways creates easier travel. We refer to this as *rewriting the neural architecture.*

Fortunately, you can rewrite the neural architecture in your stress response system, even if you've had the same responses to situations multiple times. Once the research team at the Institute of HeartMath learned how the brain and the heart were interacting, we saw the potential for grooving new pathways using the "master pendulum." With a little practice, you can change your internal habits.

Here's a story from a grateful patient, S. H., that describes her process of rewriting.

For the past five years, every time I went to the doctor my blood pressure was elevated. I passed it off as white coat syndrome. Last time I went to the doctor he said that since it was elevated every time, he would assume that I do have hypertension. I used a blood pressure monitor at home and found out that indeed my systolic blood pressure was running around 140–145. I was not able to lower it below that. My diastolic pressure was fine. I had tried to avoid facing the facts.

My doctor did some tests to rule out other problems like kidney dysfunction or salt imbalances in my system. After those came out negative, I considered that my stress level and out-of-balance emotions might be the source of my high pressure. I can be a pretty high-amp person. Then I took a little time to reflect on just this past year. I was functioning at a very high level in my job, bringing in more sales than I ever had. I remodeled and painted my home. I faced some of my biggest fears, and had some other physical challenges. I had lost two close friends to cancer. Could I possibly have reset my system to believe that stress was the norm?

A very close and respected friend gave me the advice that I would be able to calm myself and reset my system. I knew that many people had good results lowering their blood pressure using the HeartMath tools. So I set out to do it.

I began by taking short time-outs during the day to use the Quick Coherence technique. First I would tune in to how I was feeling inside. Next I would take a few seconds and tell myself I was going to calm myself. Next, I would take about twenty or thirty seconds to breathe a feeling of calm in and out of my heart. Then I recalled a time I felt very calm and peaceful inside, such as sitting on the top of a ridge with friends quietly looking out over the mountain ranges.

I have been doing this for about two weeks now. I stop and do it whenever I catch myself with too much "amp" inside, or when I have an emotional reaction to something, or catch myself holding my breath. By being more conscious all day long as to whether I was relaxed or not, I discovered that I was moving too fast and out of sync.

After one week, I began to get some readings between 120 and 138, mostly in the lower range. This gave me hope. I added two special ten- to fifteen-minute Heart Lock-In sessions [the technique you will learn in this chapter] *to my day, while listening to Doc Childre's Heart Zones music. I focus on calming myself and sending appreciation to myself for doing this and then sending appreciation to others. More and more during the day when I catch myself getting overly concerned or upset about something, I say to myself, "It's just not worth it" and do a Quick Coherence exercise.*

When I am deeply relaxed my systolic blood pressure runs lower. I am now able to actually feel inside when my blood pressure is up. I feel a nervous feeling running in my veins and it is more difficult to

*relax. So I stay with Quick Coherence, repeating the
steps, until I feel myself relax deeply.*

*I know I have to stay very diligent to reset my
system. I often wake up with the adrenaline running
in my system. But I feel there is real hope in applying
the HeartMath tools to reset this. I have made a
commitment to myself to stay very steady with my
practice.*

Heart Lock-In

The final technique you will learn in this book is called Heart
Lock-In. While there are a number of other HeartMath tools
and techniques, the use of Neutral, Quick Coherence, and
Heart Lock-In will be the most helpful to you in lowering
your blood pressure.

The Heart Lock-In technique is to be used daily, to help
sustain coherence to rewrite your pathways and make a
psychological and physiological habit out of more beneficial
responses. This technique builds on the steps that you've
already learned, with slight modification.

1. **Shift** your attention to the area of the heart and
    breathe slowly and deeply.

2. **Activate** and sustain a genuine feeling of
    appreciation or care for someone or something
    in your life.

3. **Send** these feelings of appreciation or care
    toward yourself and others.

After shifting your attention to the center of your chest,
and breathing slowly in and out through your heart, send
these feelings of appreciation or care to yourself and others.
Sending feelings may seem strange at first, but everyone

unconsciously sends feelings to their bodies and to other people all the time.

Your Energies Do Affect Others

Did you ever wonder why some people always seem to affect you negatively, while others always seem to make you feel great? Relationships between people, at home or at work, are based on the same principles of coherence and chaos. The very powerful heart signal is not only causing contractions in your heart muscle. That big signal is doing lots of things to you—physically, emotionally, and mentally, as we've seen. Remember how we discussed that the strong electromagnetic field generated by the heart can be measured well outside your body? The latest research from our laboratory has shown that these signals are also picked up by other people's nervous systems.

Your stress and negativity really do affect other people, just as your positive emotions have an effect. The Heart Lock-In technique helps you to become more conscious of this process. By learning to intentionally send positive emotions to yourself and others, you sustain coherence longer and increase its positive effect.

A good place to start step 2 is to appreciate *yourself* for a minute or two. There are probably many things about yourself that you could appreciate. Go ahead—nobody's looking. If you have trouble finding something, simply appreciate yourself for reading this book and making a sincere effort to lower your blood pressure and improve your health. You are in charge here. This isn't your doctor telling you what you have to do, or writing you a prescription. It isn't anything that's going to give you side effects (except the "side effects" of having cortical facilitation and possibly improving your health, your home life, and your work life). Now appreciate yourself for practicing these tools. You're taking the time, and doing something for yourself, as simple as it may seem.

After appreciating yourself — really feel that appreciative attitude — just shift a little and radiate that appreciation out to others. You might pick members of your family for this exercise today. Tomorrow you might pick people who have helped you out in times of need. Or your book club, or your tennis group, or people you are close to at work or at your church. Simply expand the focus of your appreciation outward from yourself to those around you.

Sustaining Coherence

Try to sustain appreciative feelings and attitudes in a Heart Lock-In for five minutes or longer. The longer you can do this and hold it, the better it is for you and your system. You're learning to sustain coherence.

Remember, if your thoughts wander or you are distracted in some other way, it's not a problem. Just go back to Heart Focus and Heart Breathing. Once you've gotten back into your heart breathing rhythm, simply return to appreciating yourself and then radiate appreciation out to your chosen group for this session.

When to Practice Heart Lock-In

Practicing the Heart Lock-In technique for ten or fifteen minutes every day — all at once, or divided into two or three sessions — helps to very quickly groove beneficial pathways driven by coherence. It's ideal to spend some time at the beginning of each day doing this, before the horns in your world start blowing, and the phone calls start pouring in, and the e-mails start flooding your in-box. Why not start the day with a coherent program playing in your system?

Most people find that doing a Heart Lock-In a couple of times a day helps to accumulate energy and recharge their emotional system. It cushions the impact of day-to-day stress and reduces energy drain. Doing a short, midday Lock-In is very effective for offsetting the feeling of afternoon drag. That drag results in less focus and motivation. It's also a time when you might be tempted to snack or grab another cup of coffee to pump up your energy level. Let Heart Lock-In reenergize your emotional system instead.

Another time to use Heart Lock-In is just before sleep. Many have found that doing the Heart Lock-In technique at this time promotes a more restful sleep and is especially helpful with insomnia.

Practicing the Heart Lock-In technique while listening to background music that lifts your spirit can increase its positive effects (McCraty et al. 1996; McCraty et al. 1998; McCraty, Atkinson, and Tomasino 2001). Coauthor Doc Childre has created two music CDs that are designed to be used with Heart Lock-In to facilitate coherence and emotional regeneration (see "Learn More About HeartMath").

Heart Lock-In helps to rewrite the old, automatic programming and to lock-in a new pattern so that when you need to quickly use Neutral or Quick Coherence in the heat of the moment, the coherent pattern and pathway becomes more accessible, and eventually preferred.

In a short while, and with some regular practice, you won't have to stop and recall all the steps of the tools. For example, with Heart Lock-In, all you'll need to remember are the key words: shift, activate, and send. Your "switch" will be readily available to you. You will find that simply shifting your attention to your heart will start the cascade of positive reactions inside, just as your old habits triggered the negative reactions.

You have control over your programming. Now have some fun and use these tools. You will be surprised to look back and see how often you were hijacked by your old responses, and how effective your new responses have become.

Chapter 11

HeartMath Studies

HeartMath began designing and delivering training programs based on these tools to corporations, health professionals, and individuals in the mid-1990s. Many companies, especially the larger ones, had begun noticing that stress was taking an increasing toll on their employees at all levels. One of the "symptoms" was the number of health care dollars being spent on stress-related complaints. Ten years later that number is much higher. The American Institute of Stress estimates that between 75 and 90 percent of visits to primary care physicians are related in some way to stress (Rosch 1991).

Another observation made by large employers was that productivity was affected by stress and stress-related illnesses. Absenteeism was much higher in workers who reported high levels of stress. Companies were beginning to realize that the stress epidemic was very costly to them.

The Institute of HeartMath has always been a data-driven organization. Our scientists and advisors felt very strongly that our interventions should be carefully monitored to validate their effectiveness and so that we could make refinements to our methods. So when we designed the first HeartMath corporate training program, which took place at

Motorola in 1995, we also designed a statistically analyzable questionnaire to measure personal and organizational stress and the symptoms and problems that went with it. Before administering this questionnaire, physiological measures were collected. Blood pressure, of course, happened to be one of them.

Early Results

Forty-eight employees at three levels within Motorola were selected to participate in a HeartMath stress-management course. Nine executives, nine software engineers, and thirty factory workers attended, but blood pressure recordings were only available in the first two groups (executives and engineers). Five of the participants were found to have hypertension.

Six months after the subjects participated in the program where they learned HeartMath tools and were encouraged (but not mandated) to practice them daily, the blood pressure readings had dropped significantly in all five of the subjects. In addition, further reductions were seen immediately after the participants were asked to practice a variation of the Quick Coherence technique while their blood pressure was being monitored.

It's important to realize that this program was not designed to lower blood pressure, but rather to give the participants tools to reduce their own levels of stress and enhance their enjoyment of work. Blood pressure was simply one of the variables being measured in the process. Follow-up testing six months later found that contentment, job satisfaction, and communication all improved in the group as a whole. Not surprisingly, feelings of tension and anxiety were reduced, as were physical symptoms of stress.

Five people with hypertension is a very small number. But in this early research study, the HeartMath team was very excited to see that blood pressure dropped significantly in each of the five participants. It was a great beginning.

We noted something else back in the mid-1990s — that people attending the corporate programs gave stress only minor acknowledgment. But as time went along and more seminars were delivered, more and more people admitted that stress was a bigger and bigger problem in both their personal lives and at work.

Shortly after this first study, the team designed another study specifically to evaluate whether Inner Quality Management, a corporate stress-management program using the HeartMath tools, could improve emotional health and reduce blood pressure in employees at a large and well-known global information technology company. The study was based on earlier observations that the HeartMath techniques had favorably altered autonomic nervous system measurements (McCraty et al. 1995; Tiller, McCraty, and Atkinson 1996), reduced cortisol levels and increased DHEA levels (McCraty et al. 1998), and enhanced immune activity (McCraty et al. 1996; Rein, Atkinson, and McCraty 1995).

Twenty-eight male and female employees of this company were assigned either to a group that received the HeartMath Inner Quality Management training, or to a control group that was waiting to be trained in these tools. The two groups had essentially the same characteristics (height, weight, gender, blood pressure levels, and whether or not medications were being taken for hypertension), though there was a slight difference in the average ages of the two groups (forty-eight in the treatment group versus forty-three in the control group).

The results of this study were also very encouraging (see figure 2). After three months, the average drop in systolic blood pressure was 10.6 points for the people who learned the HeartMath tools. The diastolic pressures dropped as well. Interestingly, both systolic and diastolic pressures also dropped by small amounts in the control group waiting for HeartMath training (McCraty, Atkinson, and Tomasino 2003). This is often seen in scientific studies. Scientists believe that when people are being paid attention to in a study, even though they are not in the "active treatment" group, changes can occur no matter what the study is measuring (blood pressure, in this case). This is precisely why it's important to have a control group in a research experiment—so the observed changes can be compared between the treated subjects and the control subjects. In this case, the diastolic pressures, even though they dropped by an average of 6.3 points in the experimental group, were not different enough from the drop seen in the controls (3.9 points) to reach statistical significance.

How does the big drop in systolic blood pressure seen in the people practicing the HeartMath tools compare to some of the other lifestyle changes that hypertensive patients are encouraged to make? A 10.6-point drop in systolic blood pressure would be equivalent to the changes expected with a forty-pound weight loss, or twice the drop expected with either a salt-restricted diet or an exercise program.

Because the study was designed to cut stress in the workplace, the researchers were also gratified that in addition to lowering blood pressure, treatment also significantly decreased depression and other symptoms of stress, and workers developed a more positive outlook about their jobs. These results point out once again that mood is highly correlated with blood pressure.

Blood Pressure Reductions in Hypertensive Individuals

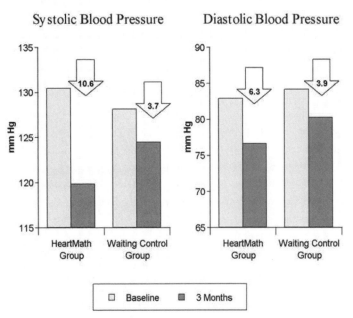

Figure 2: Systolic and diastolic blood pressure in males and females practicing HeartMath tools vs. those waiting to be trained.

Correlating Mood and Blood Pressure

In another very interesting study conducted by the National Center of Health Statistics, Centers for Disease Control and Prevention in Maryland, Dr. Bruce Jonas and his colleagues followed almost 3,000 people with normal blood pressure for up to sixteen years. They looked at both blacks and whites in two age groups (25–44 and 45–64). There was a high correlation between the development of high blood pressure in people with high levels of anxiety and depression. This study was important because it showed that people with negative emotional states (mood) are two to three times more likely to develop hypertension in the future (Jonas, Franks, and Ingram 1997). The physiology of this was discussed in the last chapter when we discussed the emotions of stress. T. M.'s story, below, is a great example.

> *T. M. is a fifty-two-year-old male executive in a high-tech company. There is a strong family history of hypertension. Since 1986, T. M. had gone to extreme measures to manage his high blood pressure — transferring to less-stressful positions, leaving his job altogether (twice), losing weight, exercising, removing salt from his diet, and growing, preparing, and canning all his own food without salt — all to no avail. An internist suspected that T. M.'s condition was anxiety related and prescribed Serzone, an antidepressant medication with antianxiety effects. Initial success was short-lived. After several months, T. M. noticed his blood pressure creeping back up until it reached an average of 170/110. T. M. attended a HeartMath seminar in the fall of 1998 and found that he could bring about profound improvements in his high blood pressure using the HeartMath tools. In a letter written in March 1999, four months after his introduction to the techniques, T. M. reported that his blood pressure readings were as low as 97/75, readings he had not seen in over twenty years. He was able to stop taking the Serzone and noted, "My family has commented that I am noticeably different, a comment I never received while using prescription medications for anxiety."*

Beyond the Corporate World

Have you ever thought that your job must be the most stressful one on earth? Oddly enough, you are not alone. The Institute of HeartMath completed a fascinating study of correctional officers in three prison facilities (McCraty et al. 2003). (Still think your job is the most stressful?)

The study enrolled eighty-eight officers and split them into two groups. The control group waited for the program, while the study group learned about health risk factors and attended a seminar on stress management using the HeartMath tools. Follow-up took place after three months.

Although the numbers were relatively small and the follow-up period was short, the biggest problem with this study was that the study group and the controls were all in the workplace together. On top of that, some of the members of the study group were married to members of the control group waiting to take the course later, so there was quite a bit of crosstalk between groups.

Despite these problems, which made the statistical comparison between groups more difficult, this study made some fascinating observations. After three months, the officers reported the following changes:

- decreased stress
- decreased anger
- decreased fatigue
- decreased hostility
- decreased impatience
- decreased overall psychological distress

- increased goal clarity
- increased motivation
- increased productivity
- increased gratitude
- increased positive outlook
- increased perceived managerial support

But what about *blood pressure*? Both their systolic and diastolic pressures fell significantly. As seen in figure 3, significant reductions were also seen in the following:

- Heart rate

- Blood glucose

- Total cholesterol

- LDL (bad) cholesterol

- Total/HDL cholesterol ratio

Taken together, the government organization that commissioned the study determined that all of these improvements added up to a projected healthcare savings of about $700 per employee per year.

HeartMath in Health Care

It's clear from years of experience and scientific testing that learning and practicing the HeartMath tools can make a very big difference in your life. As a cardiologist, I (Dr. Bruce Wilson) had my first experience with HeartMath in the context of finding a scientifically based program of stress reduction for patients with heart disease.

After initially resisting the offer to attend a program, I found myself riveted to my chair back in 1997 as Dr. McCraty spoke about the original research done at HeartMath. The observations about the very powerful communication between the heart and the brain nearly knocked me off my seat. Like other physicians, I was taught throughout my medical education to doubt everything that passed in front of me. That's a good thing, for the most part, because it helps doctors guide their patients to interventions that are based on hard evidence.

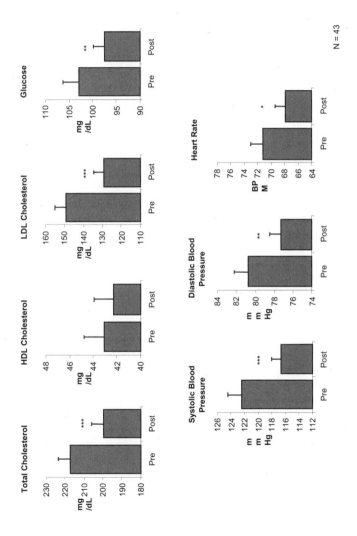

Figure 3: Physiological Measures of Experimental Group Before and After Intervention

But there I sat, a heart doctor who had passed all the tests along the way, having my nearly-etched-in-stone model of how the heart and brain worked turned literally upside down.

I was fascinated by how the heart rhythm shifts into the coherent state when you feel positive emotions, such as appreciation or care. I immediately saw how this coherent state would be important for my patients, because their cardiovascular systems would operate much more efficiently. Getting synchronization between all systems in the body makes them all more efficient, using less energy to accomplish more. That's really what the word "efficiency" means.

The early HeartMath studies told me that just shifting into this state of coherence could reduce most people's blood pressure around eight to ten points. If they practiced regularly, they could reduce it more. I could see that by teaching my patients how to make this shift, they might not only reduce their stress, but with practice they could retrain their internal pathways so that coherence would become more familiar to their hearts and brains. This in turn might very well return the set point or thermostat that controls their blood pressure to more normal baseline levels and, potentially, lead to long-term reductions in their blood pressure readings.

As I mentioned in the introduction, it wasn't long before my thoughts turned to helping the caregivers in hospitals as well. Their own stress levels often get in the way of giving sincere care, despite all the boxes being checked in the charts. With a lot of ingenuity and careful listening, the HeartMath team developed a Health Care Division and a program for hospitals to help nurses and other staff to manage their own stress better and deliver care from the heart. Nurses have to have lots of brain power, too, but having reached this point in the book, you are now well aware of what happens when negative emotions and stress prevent coherence from the heart.

The Delnor Story

The first hospital to implement the HeartMath program was Delnor Hospital in Aurora, Illinois, near Chicago. That hospital is now famous for incorporating the HeartMath tools into their local culture. They were experiencing very high levels of turnover in their nursing staff—a very expensive problem. After training 400 people in their hospital in the HeartMath tools, their overall turnover ratio dropped dramatically in the first year from 27 percent to 4 percent. The nurse turnover savings alone were estimated at $880,000 in that first year. Their patient satisfaction scores improved dramatically, as did their employee satisfaction. They calculated that in that year alone, they saved over $2 million by actually influencing their internal culture with HeartMath. Tom Wright, the chief operating officer, commented, "HeartMath gave us the tools to move from required courtesy to genuine care. As a result, we have achieved our benchmarks in patient satisfaction and employee satisfaction excellence. Without HeartMath, we could not have reached our potential."

Delnor has continued to enjoy huge savings every year since having the HeartMath program in place, and has won multiple awards for it. Many other hospitals and systems have since brought this program to their employees and have not only saved millions of dollars, but changed the culture of care from the heart up, not from the top down.

HRV Feedback Tools

Many health care providers have learned of the HeartMath program and have incorporated it into their practices. Physicians, chiropractors, psychologists, biofeedback experts, and others have been trained to teach the tools using a computer-based HRV software program. This technology displays the HRV (heart rate variability) pattern in real time through the use of a finger sensor or an ear sensor. In addition to many other features, it feeds back to the learner how coherent the heart signal is in many different ways. This technology, in fact, was used by many of the people with high blood pressure who were mentioned in the stories a little earlier, to help with their HeartMath tool practice.

Many health care providers now use HeartMath tools along with the HRV feedback technology with patients having many different health issues, both physical and emotional. One therapist has been able to get over 400 children off drugs for ADD/ADHD. There are many success stories from learning to increase and sustain coherence levels.

Creative Stress

Stress, at times, can make some people more productive. It can motivate them—for awhile—until they lose focus and their energy drops. But when stressful attitudes and feelings continue day after day, month after month, they take a toll. It's the unmanaged stress reactions to people, issues, and situations that contribute to unhappiness, strained relationships, accelerated aging, and physical diseases. Blood pressure happens to be just one of the diseases, and a very common one at that.

The practice of HeartMath tools has helped people all around the globe. You have now seen the results: People who use the HeartMath techniques have gained an understanding about how they react to small or annoying events and changed their responses. This practice has helped them to then change their responses to bigger events. They have learned that the ability to throw their master switch to coherence is quite simple, and therefore quite powerful. The benefits are essentially endless.

The big picture is that you can learn to bring yourself less stress and become more efficient and effective at the same time. You can choose how you wish to respond to situations in life. In doing so, you may very well improve your blood pressure. And there are no side effects.

Chapter 12

The End Is Just the Beginning

You undoubtedly purchased this book because you wanted to do something about your blood pressure. Whether you're the type who doesn't like the idea of taking pills and medications, or you want to do something for yourself in addition to taking meds, you were interested enough to open these pages and learn about the HeartMath program and its tools.

You joined us on a journey. You learned a fair amount about blood pressure along the way, such as the fact that 90 to 95 percent of hypertension is termed "essential" hypertension, meaning without a known cause. Lots of things can contribute to high blood pressure, but only 5 to 10 percent of the time can doctors identify a specific physical problem causing it.

You were guided along a brief tour of the complexities of the human body. You saw how the kidneys react to hormones from the adrenal glands and make their own blood pressure–raising substance when blood pressure drops or when they are simply fooled into thinking the pressure is low.

You had a review of pharmacology, and saw how the different types of medications are supposed to lower your blood pressure. We say "supposed to" because sometimes they don't—and they may have side effects. Almost everybody's blood pressure can be returned to the normal range, given enough time, effort, and patience on the part of both the patient and the physician, but it's not always a smooth ride. You also read about what happens when hypertension is not adequately treated.

But then another view began to unfold. You had a glimpse into the physiological world of stress and how it affects your entire system. You learned that your brain is a pattern-matching organ and that events in your environment, even though they may not threaten your survival, can trip the alarm system just as life-threatening situations do. Your emotional responses are an integral part of the stress response, and begin to form patterns that, when reinforced over and over, can become habitual. That patterned stress response with all of its 1,400 chemical reactions can poison your system in many ways, not the least of which is to give you hypertension.

Stress is becoming an epidemic all over the world: Reporting on the results of a poll conducted by the American Psychological Association, Kate Schuler wrote in an article for *USA Today* on February 23, 2006, that about half of the respondents said they were worried about levels of stress in their lives, and only about half of those who were concerned were taking steps to deal with that stress. People may attend seminars or buy books or watch infomercials that tell them to change their diets or exercise more, but they're often too stressed-out to follow through. They seek comfort in things that only compound the problem (eating, drinking, smoking, drugs). Going on vacation, going to church, attending a yoga class, or learning to meditate can all be helpful, but they all have to be done . . . later. And the stress returns when they walk back through the door to work or home.

The HeartMath tools you learned in this book have two very attractive characteristics: They are easy to learn, and they work. This is possible because new research has shown that the heart is not just a pump — it's an extremely powerful signal generator that eclipses the power of the brain signals many times over. Instead of arguing with those little, tiny brain waves, HeartMath enables people to naturally engage the heart, and coax it into sending coherence throughout the system, markedly altering brain function and stopping the toxic stress response in its tracks.

The world has become a complicated place, and it's not likely to become less complicated. There is no pill, or machine, or exercise program, or lottery ticket that will wipe stress overload off the map.

Over 50,000 people on five continents have learned the HeartMath tools. They have learned, quite literally, to go to their hearts to manage their emotions and gain new perspectives. Because the tools are so simple and easy to learn, many are quite surprised to see themselves coming up with new perceptions and answers. This is why we use the term "heart intelligence." The trick, once these tools are learned, is to practice going to the heart to achieve coherence *before* the breaking point in order to maintain physical and emotional health . . . and lower your blood pressure.

Just as with all the antihypertensive medications, there is no guarantee that your blood pressure will normalize if you practice and use these tools. But there aren't any side effects except being emotionally and physically healthier, and having the ability to respond differently to the ever more complex world around you.

There are a number of other HeartMath tools and applications. People in individual, corporate, health care, and education programs have learned a host of simple techniques since the early '90s. As a side effect, there was a surprising drop in blood pressure in those who used and practiced the HeartMath tools. That's eventually how this book came to be written. Having high blood pressure is a wonderful reason for you to have found HeartMath. Learning small, simple techniques to activate your heart intelligence can make so much difference in negotiating the stress out of your system.

Start practicing these heart techniques with the small stresses—those tiny things that get to you—the short traffic jam, the empty paper tray in the copier, the long line at the grocery store. Once you get a little practice engaging your heart to reprogram your responses, move up to your bigger stresses and see if you don't also see them from a different angle—a wider perspective. If you can't solve or relieve a problem completely, and often you can't, you can at least take some of the emotional charge out of it. Over time, you'll be surprised to see a lot of problems improve without you having wasted or drained your energy in the process. You'll see that it's the significance that you assign to any issue that ramps up your stress response until the response is actually bigger than the issue itself. These tools, by changing brain function at the highest level, allow you to see the problems in a different light, and often from another angle, which will ultimately lessen their significance. This is done by first changing the heart. As the saying goes, "A change of heart changes everything."

Congratulations. You have taken some personal responsibility. It all started with your blood pressure. But you've walked through a bigger door—welcome.

APPENDIX

Classes of Drugs Used to Treat Hypertension

TABLE I: Diuretics

Generic Name	*Trade Name*
Bumetanide	Bumex
Chlorthalidone	Hygroton
Ethacrynic acid	Edecrin
Furosemide	Lasix
Hydrochlorothiazide (HCTZ)	HydroDIURIL, Microzide
Indapamide	Lozol
Metolazone	Zaroxolyn, Mykrox
Torsemide	Demadex

TABLE II: Beta-blockers

Generic Name	*Trade Name*
Acebutolol	Sectral
Atenolol	Tenormin
Carvedilol	Coreg
Labetalol	Normodyne, Trandate
Metoprolol	Lopressor, Toprol
Nadolol	Corgard
Pindolol	Visken
Propranolol	Inderal

TABLE III: ACE inhibitors/ARBs

Generic Name	*Trade Name*

ACE Inhibitors

Generic Name	Trade Name
Benazepril	Lotensin
Captopril	Capoten
Enalapril	Vasotec
Fosinopril	Monopril
Moexipril	Univasc
Perindopril	Aceon
Quinapril	Accupril
Ramipril	Altace
Trandolapril	Mavik

ARBs

Generic Name	Trade Name
Candesartan	Atacand
Eprosartan	Teveten
Irbesartan	Avapro
Losartan	Cozaar
Olmesartan	Benicar
Telmisartan	Micardis
Valsartan	Diovan

TABLE IV: Calcium channel blockers

Generic Name	*Trade Name*
Amlodipine	Norvasc
Diltiazem	Cardizem, Tiazac
Felodipine	Plendil
Nicardipine	Cardene
Nifedipine	Procardia, Adalat
Verapamil	Calan, Isoptin, Verelan

TABLE V: Aldosterone blockers

Generic Name	*Trade Name*
Eplerenone	Inspra
Spironolactone	Aldactone

TABLE VI: Alpha blockers

Generic Name	*Trade Name*
Doxazosin	Cardura
Prazosin	Minipress
Terazosin	Hytrin

TABLE VII: Sympatholytic drugs

Generic Name	*Trade Name*
Clonidine	Catapres
Guanabenz	Wytensin
Methyldopa	Aldomet

TABLE VIII: Direct vasodilators

Generic Name	*Trade Name*
Hydralazine	Apresoline
Minoxidil	Loniten

Learn More About HeartMath

Explore other HeartMath books, learning programs, music, software, seminars, and professional training to reinforce and advance what you've learned in this book. More details can be found online at *www.heartmath.com.*

Books and Learning Programs

Childre, Doc and Deborah Rozman. 2006. *Transforming Anxiety: the HeartMath Solution for Overcoming Fear and Worry and Creating Serenity.* Oakland, CA: New Harbinger Publications, Inc.

Childre, Doc and Deborah Rozman. 2005. *Transforming Stress: The HeartMath Solution for Relieving Worry, Fatigue, and Tension.* Oakland, CA: New Harbinger Publications, Inc.

Childre, Doc and Deborah Rozman. 2003. *Transforming Anger: The HeartMath Solution for Letting Go of Rage, Frustration, and Irritation.* Oakland, CA: New Harbinger Publications, Inc.

Childre, Doc, and Howard Martin. 1999. *The HeartMath Solution.* San Francisco: HarperSanFrancisco.

Childre, Doc, and Bruce Cryer. 2000. *From Chaos to Coherence: The Power to Change Performance.* Boulder Creek, CA: Planetary Publications.

From Chaos to Coherence (CD-ROM). Boulder Creek, CA: HeartMath LLC and Knowledgebuilder.com.

Childre, Doc. 1998. *Freeze-Frame: A Scientifically Proven Technique for Clear Decision Making and Improved Health.* Boulder Creek, CA: Planetary Publications.

Childre, Doc. 1992. *The How To Book of Teen Self Discovery.* Boulder Creek, CA: Planetary Publications.

Music by Doc Childre

These recordings are scientifically designed to enhance the practice of HeartMath techniques and tools.

Heart Zones. Planetary Publications.

Speed of Balance. Planetary Publications.

Quiet Joy. Planetary Publications.

emWave PC™

Powered Stress Relief System (formerly known as the Freeze-Framer®)

The emWave PC is a patented interactive learning system with a heart rhythm monitor and pulse sensor. This software-based program allows you to observe your heart rhythms in real time and assists you in increasing coherence to reduce stress and improve health and performance

emWave™ Personal Stress Reliever®

emWave Personal Stress Reliever represents a breakthrough in stress reduction technology. This stress reliever helps to build a cushion between you and day-to-day stress, thereby enhancing energy and performance. This mobile device weighs just 2.2 ounces and is small enough to fit in your purse or pocket, so you can take it with you and use it anytime, anywhere.

emTech™ Media Products

The emTechT products were created by utilizing information from a variety of HeartMath sources. They offer some of the best subject-specific information found in the HeartMath System, and are available as e-booklets, audio programs and interactive learning modules.

Test Edge™ Interactive CD-ROM - Grades 9-12 and above

This unique interactive learning program helps students balance their mental and emotional systems, which is critical for successful learning and test taking. Without this balance, feelings of anxiety and fear jam the connection between what students really know and what they can actually express, especially while taking tests.

The TestEdge practices are also designed to help students deal with the emotions they carry into the classroom stemming from peer pressure overload and problems at home, which can slow or block learning.

HeartMath Seminars and Training

HeartMath provides world-class training programs for organizations, hospitals, health care providers, and individuals. HeartMath training is available through on-site programs for organizations and through sponsored workshops, seminars, and conference presentations.

Licensing and Certification: Training to Become a One-on-One Provider

HeartMath offers licensing and certification to health care providers, coaches, and consultants wanting to use HeartMath tools and technologies as part of the services they provide to clients in a one-on-one professional model.

Licensing and Certification: "Train the Trainer" Programs for Organizations

HeartMath offers licensing and training to organizations wanting to make the HeartMath tools and technologies a part of their offerings to internal customers, employees, or members.

For information on products, seminars, and workshops, call (800) 450-9111, e-mail *info@heartmath.com*, visit the Web site at *www.heartmath.com*, or write to: HeartMath, 14700 West Park Avenue, Boulder Creek, CA 95006.

Research and Education

The Institute of HeartMath (IHM) is a nonprofit research and education organization dedicated to understanding emotions and the role of the heart in learning, performance, and well-being. IHM offers programs for use in educational and classroom settings, including:

- *TestEdge* programs for improving academic performance and test scores

- *Resiliency* programs for teachers, administrators, and principals

- *Emotional Security Tool Kit for Children and Teens*, which includes HeartMath techniques to reduce anger, worry, and anxiety, adapted for children ages two to eighteen, available for free at *www.heartmath.org*

For information about Institute of HeartMath research initiatives and education programs, corporate sponsorship, donations, or endowments, please call (831) 338-8500, e-mail *info@heartmath.org*, visit the Web site at *www.heartmath.org*, or write to: Institute of HeartMath, 14700 West Park Avenue, Boulder Creek, CA 95006.

References

Anderson, S. 2003. Pathogenesis of hypertensive renal damage. In *Hypertension Primer*, 3rd ed., ed. J. Izzo Jr. and H. Black. Dallas: Lippincott, Williams and Wilkins.

Appel, L. J., T. J. Moore, E. Obarzamek, W. M. Vollmer, L. P. Svetkey, F. M. Sacks, G. A. Bray, T. M. Vogt, J. A. Cutler, M. M. Windhauser, P.-H. Lin, and N. Karanja. 1997. A clinical trial of the effects of dietary patterns on blood pressure: Results from the Dietary Approaches to Stop Hypertension (DASH) trail. *New England Journal of Medicine* 336(16):1117–24.

Bruenn, H. 1970. Clinical notes on the illness and death of President Franklin Delano Roosevelt. *Annals of Internal Medicine* 72:579–91.

Cameron, O. 2002. *Visceral Sensory Neuroscience: Introception.* New York: Oxford University Press.

Chobanian, A. V., G. H. Bakris, H. R. Black, W. Cushman, L. Green, J. Izzo, D. Jones, B. J. Materson, S. Oparil, J. T. Wright Jr., and E. J. Rocella. 2003. Seventh report of the Joint National Committee on Prevention, Detection, and Treatment of High Blood Pressure. *Hypertension* 42:1206–52.

Fields, L. E., V. L. Burt, J. A. Cutler, E. Rocella, and P. Sorlie. 2004. The burden of adult hypertension in the United States 1999 to 2000: A rising tide. *Hypertension* 44:398–404.

Frysinger, R., and R. Harper. 1990. Cardiac and respiratory correlations with unit discharge in epileptic human temporal lobe. *Epilepsia* 31:162–71.

Hawkley, L., C. Masi, J. Berry, and J. Cacioppo. 2006. Loneliness is a unique predictor of age-related difference in systolic blood pressure. *Psychology and Aging* 21:152–64.

Hay, J. 1931. The significance of a raised blood pressure. *British Medical Journal* 2:43–47.

Heistad, D., W. Lawton, and W. Talman. 2003. Pathogenesis of acute hypertensive encephalopathy. In *Hypertension Primer*, 3rd ed., ed J. Izzo Jr. and H. Black. Dallas: Lippincott, Williams and Wilkins.

Hershey, L. 2003. Pathogenesis of mild cognitive impairment and mixed dementia. In *Hypertension Primer*, 3rd ed., ed. J. Izzo Jr. and H. Black. Dallas: Lippincott, Williams and Wilkins.

Jonas, B., P. Franks, and D. Ingram. 1997. Are symptoms of anxiety and depression risk factors for hypertension? Longitudinal evidence from the National Health and Nutrition Examination Survey I Epidemiologic Follow-up Study. *Archives of Family Medicine* 6:43–49.

Lehrer, P., E. Vaschillo, B. Vaschillo, S. Lu, D. Eckberg, R. Edelberg, W. Shih, Y. Lin, T. A. Kuusela, K. U. Tahvanainen, and R. M. Hamer. 2003. Heart rate variability biofeedback increases baroreflex gain and peak expiratory flow. *Psychosomatic Medicine* 65(5):796–805.

McCraty, R. 2006. Emotional stress, positive emotions, and psychophysiological coherence. In *Stress in Health and Disease*, ed. B. Arnetz and R. Ekman, 4–5. Weinheim: Wiley-VCH.

McCraty, R., M. Atkinson, L. Lipsenthal, and L. Arguelles. 2003. *Impact of the Power to Change Performance Program on Stress and Health Risks in Correctional Officers.* Boulder Creek, CA: HeartMath Research Center, Institute of HeartMath, Publication No. 03-014.

McCraty, R., M. Atkinson, G. Rein, and A. Watkins. 1996. Music enhances the effect of positive emotional states on salivary IgA. *Stress Medicine* 12:167–75.

McCraty, R., M. Atkinson, W. Tiller, G. Rein, and A. Watkins. 1995. The effects of emotions on short-term power spectrum analysis of heart rate variability. *American Journal of Cardiology* 76:1089–93.

McCraty, R., M. Atkinson, and D. Tomasino. 2001. *Science of the Heart: Exploring the Role of the Heart in Human Performance.* Boulder Creek, CA: HeartMath Research Center, Institute of HeartMath, Publication No. 01-001.

– – –. 2003. Impact of a workplace stress reduction program on blood pressure and emotional health in hypertensive employees. *Journal of Alternative and Complementary Medicine* 9(3):355–69.

McCraty, R., B. Barrios-Choplin, D. Rozman, M. Atkinson, and A. Watkins. 1998. The impact of a new emotional self-management program on stress, emotions, heart rate variablility, DHEA and cortisol. *Integrative Physiological and Behavioral Science* 33:151–70.

Newcomer, J., S. Craft, T. Hershey, K. Askius, and M. Bardgett. 1994. Glucocorticoid induced impairment in declarative memory performance in adult humans. *Journal of Neuroscience* 14(4):2047–53.

Papademitriou, V., D. Sica, and J. Izzo Jr. 2003. Thiazide and loop diuretics. In *Hypertension Primer*, 3rd ed., ed. J. Izzo Jr. and H. Black. Dallas: Lippincott, Williams and Wilkins.

Pribram, K., and F. Melges. 1969. Psychophysiological basis of emotion. In *Handbook of Clinical Neurology*, ed. P. Vinken and G. Bruyn, 316–49. Amsterdam: North-Holland Publishing Company.

Rein, G., M. Atkinson, and R. McCraty. 1995. The physiological effects of compassion and anger. *Journal of Advances in Medicine* 8:87–105.

Rosch, P. J. 1991. Job stress: America's leading adult health problem. *USA Magazine,* May.

Sandman, C., B. Walker, and C. Berka. 1982. Influence of afferent cardiovascular feedback on behavior and the cortical evoked potential. In *Perspectives in Cardiovascular Psychophysiology*, ed. J. Cacioppo and R. Petty, 189–222. New York: Guilford Press.

Sapolsky, R. 1998. *Why Zebras Don't Get Ulcers*. New York: W. H. Freeman and Company.

Schuler, K. 2006. Only Half of Worried Americans Try to Manage Their Stress. *USA Today*, February 23.

Scott, R. W. 1946. Clinical blood pressure. In *Practice of Medicine*, ed. F. Tice. Hagerstown, MD: W. F. Prior.

Sever, P., D. Gordon, W. Pert, and P. Beighton. 1980. Blood pressure and its correlates in urban and tribal Africa. *Lancet* 2(8185):60–64.

Stein, P., P. Domitrovich, H. Huikuri, R. Kleiger, and CAST Investigators. 2005. Traditional and nonlinear heart rate variability are each independently associated with mortality after myocardial infarction. *Journal of Cardiovascular Electrophysiology* 16(1):21–23.

Thomson, W. 1997. A Change of Heart. *Natural Health Magazine*, September-October.

Thorogood, M., M. Hillsdon, and C. Summerbell. 2003. Changing behaviour. *Clinical Evidence* 10:95–117.

Tiller, W., R. McCraty, and M. Atkinson. 1996. Cardiac coherence: A new, noninvasive measure of autonomic nervous system order. *Alternative Therapies in Health and Medicine* 2:52–65.

van der Molen, M., R. Somsen, and J. Orlebeke. 1985. The rhythm of the heart beat in information processing. In *Advances in Psychophysiology*, vol. 1., ed. P. Ackles, J. Jennings, and M. Coles, 1–88. London: JAI Press.

Winkelmayer, W., M. Stampfer, W. Willett, and G. Curhan. 2005. Habitual coffee intake and the risk of hypertension in women. *Journal of the American Medical Association* 294(18):2330–2335.

Bruce C. Wilson, MD, FACC, was director of acute cardiac care at the University of Minnesota before going to the University of Pittsburgh to direct the University of Pittsburgh Heart Institute. In 1991 he returned to his hometown of Milwaukee, WI, where he started a private practice in cardiology, and was chief of cardiology and director of medical education at Columbia Hospital. He is clinical associate professor of medicine at the Medical College of Wisconsin, and has won numerous teaching awards throughout his career. Dr. Wilson has been giving lectures and teaching seminars on the HeartMath tools for stress reduction and better health since 1997, and helped develop their health care division.

Doc Childre is the founder and chairman of the scientific advisory board of the Institute of HeartMath, the chairman of HeartMath, LLC, and the chairman and co-CEO of Quantum Intech. He is the author of eight books and a consultant to business leaders, scientists, educators, and the entertainment industry on Intui-Technology®. His HeartMath System and proprietary heart rhythm technologies for coherence building, called **Freeze-Framer**® and **emWave**® **Personal Stress Reliever**®, have been reported on by Newsweek.com, *USA Today,* NBC's *Today Show,* ABC's *Good Morning America,* ABC's *World News Tonight, CNN Headline News,* CNN.com, CNN Lou Dobbs, the *Wall Street Journal,* the *Harvard Business Review, The Economist's Intelligent Life, Business 2.0, Modern Health Care, Health Leaders, Prevention, Self, Natural Health, Alternative Medicine, Psychology Today,* PGA.com, *Golf* magazine, *Golf Illustrated, Allure, Cosmopolitan, FIRST for Women, Woman's World, New Woman, GQ* magazine, *Men's Health, Men's Fitness,* the *Los Angeles Times,* the *San Francisco Chronicle,* the *San Jose Mercury News,* and numerous other publications around the world.

more powerful HeartMath® tools for change
from new**harbinger**publications

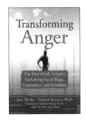

TRANSFORMING ANGER
The HeartMath® Solution for Letting Go
of Rage, Frustration, and Irritation

$12.95 • Item Code: 352X

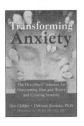

TRANSFORMING ANXIETY
The HeartMath® Solution for Overcoming
Fear and Worry and Creating Security

$12.95 • Item Code: 4445

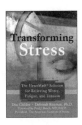

TRANSFORMING STRESS
The HeartMath® Solution for Relieving
Worry, Fatigue, and Tension

$12.95 • Item Code: 397X

available from new**harbinger**publications
and fine booksellers everywhere

To order, call toll free **1-800-748-6273** or visit our online bookstore at **www.newharbinger.com**
(V, MC, AMEX • prices subject to change without notice)